Towards a Sociology of Health Discourse in Africa

Jimoh Amzat · Oliver Razum

Towards a Sociology of Health Discourse in Africa

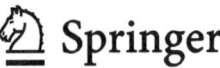 Springer

Jimoh Amzat
Department of Sociology
Usmanu Danfodiyo University
Sokoto
Nigeria

Oliver Razum
Faculty of Health Sciences
University of Bielefeld
Bielefeld
Germany

ISBN 978-3-319-61671-1   ISBN 978-3-319-61672-8 (eBook)
DOI 10.1007/978-3-319-61672-8

Library of Congress Control Number: 2017949444

Printed on acid-free paper

This Springer imprint is published by Springer Nature
The registered company is Springer International Publishing AG
The registered company address is: Gewerbestrasse 11, 6330 Cham, Switzerland

Preface

Towards a Sociology of Health Discourse in Africa is about fundamental discourses relating to health in Africa. It arises out of the consequences of endemic diseases in Africa. This book aims to identify, explain and illustrate the African-specific contexts, challenges and efforts to combat these diseases. This "discourse of disease" is part of a comprehensive sociological discourse on health in Africa and it provides a framework for students and healthcare practitioners to grasp core issues and contexts of the states of health and healthcare in Africa. What sets this volume apart is that this book is a comparative analysis of African contexts of health, but it does not ignore the global contexts of health within which Africa exists. In other words, the book presents a macroanalytic approach to health in Africa, framed around significant issues. This book is both philosophical and practical and aimed at a wide audience who may better appreciate the social dimensions of health in Africa.

Africa still battles with basic health issues including many communicable diseases such as TB and HIV/AIDS. The continent suffers from a vulnerability complex, made manifest in and through underdevelopment, global health inequalities and health system failures including inadequate infrastructure and poor health care delivery. The uniquely African issues resulting from this complex and its contexts, risks and networks of operation require critical analyses particularly in the following areas: health and healthcare delivery, the right and access to healthcare (see Chap. 2), cultural notions of health (see Chap. 5), traditional medicine in Africa (see Chap. 6), health financing and insurance (see Chap. 4), and health delivery systems such as socialist, capitalist-cum-neoliberal and two-tier systems (see Chap. 3). This book evaluates the different challenges and solutions found in contemporary healthcare in Africa and assesses how healthcare systems arise from specific political, historical, cultural and socio-economic traditions. This book will also examine African contexts of rural health (see Chap. 8), nomadic pastoralism (see Chap. 9) and healthcare emergencies (see Chap. 10). This book uses such contexts as case studies to illustrate various African policy imperatives around health and healthcare.

This book aims to broaden the readers' understanding of health issues in Africa. Through a series of comparative analyses, this book examines Africa-specific healthcare challenges and effective best practices. This book will further develop the discipline of sociology of health in Africa. As such, this book will serve as a key text in the development of the African context of healthcare discourses.

Acknowledgements

This is to acknowledge the Alexander von Humboldt Foundation for providing a renewed research fellowship to Jimoh Amzat through which this book was written and the host institution, University of Bielefeld, School of Public Health, for providing a supportive academic environment.

Contents

List of Figures

List of Tables

List of Boxes

Chapter 1
Key Concepts in Healthcare Delivery

1.1 Introduction

The field of healthcare delivery encompasses a number of concepts, including definitions of health, health systems, access to health and universal healthcare. This first chapter will examine these concepts, with the aim of setting up the background and the basis for further discussions in subsequent chapters. The starting point is the definition of health, which recently has become a subject of contention. Some scholars have called for a modification or reconsideration of the WHO definition, especially in light of current developments, particularly the worldwide rising burden of chronic diseases. As will be examined later, some alternative definitions have been proposed, which also are not free from criticisms. Creating "access to health" has been a fundamental concern of every nation, but the definition of "access to health" remains elusive. The concept of access to health is also examined focusing on its five major dimensions.

In addition to creating access to health, achieving universal health care (UHC) has been a major health goal for some decades now. "Health for all by year 2000" was a policy challenge which, unfortunately, was not met in most countries. Following limited success with the Millennial Development Goals (MDGs), the world has shifted to Global Goals and a renewed commitment to UHC. The concept of UHC is examined in this chapter with its three major components. The last concept examined here is health systems, comprised of six major building blocks including health workforce, health financing, health information, governance and leadership, medical technologies and service delivery.

1.2 What is Health?

Health can be defined in a variety of ways, but the WHO definition provides an important basis for the discussion of health and for subsequent definitions. According to the WHO, health is "a state of complete physical, mental and social well-being and

© Springer International Publishing AG 2018
J. Amzat, O. Razum, *Towards a Sociology of Health Discourse in Africa*,
DOI 10.1007/978-3-319-61672-8_1

not merely the absence of disease or infirmity" (WHO, 1946). Since its introduction in 1946, this has continued to be the most widely used definition of health in health-related literatures. Its strength lies in its inclusion of three core dimensions of health: physical, mental and social. The physical dimension refers to the proper functioning of the physiological or biological components: All of the bodies cells, tissues and organs must be functioning to ensure the survival of the organism. If any part of the body is malfunctioning, it means that the person is not healthy. The mental dimension has to do with the consciousness of the individual—consciousness devoid of illusions and characterized with a good sense of judgment and coherence, and with the absence of mental disorder or illness (whether organic or inorganic). The social dimension refers to an individual's capacity to interact with others in the society. It deals with social life and social attributes that affect morbidity and mortality.

The WHO definition combines these significant aspects to describe health and it further stipulates that it is not merely the absence of diseases or infirmity. This last aspect is also substantial. It goes beyond the germ theory of disease, which specifies that there must be a definite pathology, organic damage, or foreign antigens to establish a disease. Thus, according to the WHO definition, it is possible to be unhealthy even in the absence of those antigens. This connotes that while health is a matter involving the germ theory, other perspectives are also significant in conceptualizing or describing health. It signifies the multi-causality of health—that is, a combination of factors, some beyond the biomedical factors to include sociogenic and psychogenic factors. This multi-perspectivity is the major strength of the WHO definition of health. However, despite these strengths, the definition has been heavily criticized based on certain issues, which will be highlighted in the next section.

1.2.1 Specific Criticisms of the WHO Definition of Health

Many scholars (including Saracci, 1997; Bircher, 2005; Üstün & Jakob, 2005; Sartorius, 2006; Jadad & O'Grady, 2008; Godlee, 2011; Huber et al., 2011) have scrutinized the WHO definition of health and have pointed out a number of shortcomings. They believe these shortcomings warrant at least a modification of, if not an alternative to, the WHO definition of health. Some of the criticisms include:

1. Health is not absolute: it is generally observed that by using the word "complete," WHO is aiming for a utopian physical, social and mental health status. Such perfection is rare, if not impossible, and therefore the definition presents health as a state that is not attainable.

2. It contributes to the rising medicalization: it is also argued that by having a very broad scope, the WHO definition creates room for "everything and anything" to be defined as health issues or requiring medical attention. Medicalization is the increasing incorporation of health issues into medicine, some of which are unnecessary. Even social issues are increasingly medicalized, and there has been a proliferation of drugs for "anything and everything." In this way, the

WHO definition contributes to the medicalization of society as more and more human characteristics are recruited as risk factors for disease (Godlee, 2011) or earmarked for medical intervention.

3. It is less considerate of chronic disease: going strictly by the WHO definition, people living with chronic diseases are not healthy, as they embody, at any point in time, some form of physiological malfunctioning with, which they need to live and manage. The ability to cope with these physiological challenges is underappreciated. Huber et al. (2011) specifically stated that the definition of health as a complete state of wellbeing is no longer apt, due to the rising global burden of chronic diseases. It has further been observed that when the WHO definition was formulated, acute diseases constituted the major disease burden. With the disease pattern having shifted considerably to non-communicable diseases, the WHO definition needs reconsideration.

4. It is not measurable: the definition is vague and elusive, and therefore difficult to operationalize. As a working definition, it is hard to set out objective indicators to measure health as currently defined by WHO because of the various dimensions and its holistic stance. For Saracci (1997), what accounts for the operational/measurement problem is the widening of health to the psychological and the social dimension.

1.2.2 Alternative Definitions of Health

A number of scholars (including Bircher, 2005 and Huber et al., 2011) have provided alternative definitions of health. This section will briefly examine three holistic alternative definitions. Bircher (2005, p. 336) defined health as "a dynamic state of wellbeing characterized by a physical, mental and social potential, which satisfies the demands of a life commensurate with age, culture, and personal responsibility." As with the WHO definition, even without the word "complete," this definition also considers all three dimensions (bio-psycho-social) found in the WHO definition. The Bircher definition stipulates "potentials" instead of a "a complete state," and further clarifies that if the potential is insufficient to satisfy these demands, the state is disease.

Bircher goes on to explain that apart from children who are totally dependent on care, adults are generally in control of their health. The capacity for such control varies dramatically across the life cycle, however. Thus, illness and frailty of age increase against the level of dependence (Bircher, 2005, p. 336). In this way, the ability to fulfill life potentials and challenges defines health, and the inability to cope is a sign of ill-health. This conforms, for the most part, to the social model of health, which stresses the fulfillment of social roles in society. For instance, Parsons (1972) defined health as "the state of optimum capacity of an individual for the effective performance of the roles and tasks for which he has been socialized." According to this definition, the capacity to meet role expectations is identical to meeting life potentials, which are affected by biologically given and personally acquired partial potentials (Bircher, 2005). The potentials can be subdivided into biological (physiological endowments, such as brain, and eyes), and social (personally acquired through society, including skills, education, language). Therefore, both biological and social capabilities, including the demands of life, interact to influence the health status of an individual.

Furthermore, it is observed that although the two partial potentials (bio-social) are not directly comparable, one can complement the other. According to Bircher (2005), the relationship between the total potential and demands of life determines whether an individual is healthy or diseased. It is ill-health when the demands outweigh the potential while it is health when the potential outweighs or is equal to the demands. Invariably, those who are able to meet daily demands and roles in the society are regarded as healthy. One of the major strengths of this definition is the potential to offer yardsticks or indicators for measuring health. It also significantly takes into account the possibility of chronic disease, dwindling capacity due to ageing, and the relative social roles based on culture. The definition also notes that the demands of life vary from individual to individual due to relative life aspirations, at least apart from general or normal life demands.

The Bircher's definition, however, neglects the possibility of negative potentials, which could be detrimental to the society. In this instance, experience of socio-psychological fixation in the process of socialization might imply negative potentials. Also, culture is relative and complex. It is not everything that is cultural can be medically acceptable or considered healthy. For instance, Efik culture views fatness as a mark of beauty, hence, the Efik people practice forced fattening of slim women (Simmons, 1998). There are a number of cultural precepts, which individuals have been socialized to accept and conform with, which might have negative potentials or roles for well-being.

In another vein, Huber et al. (2011) defined "health as the ability to adapt and self-manage in the face of social, physical, and emotional challenges." As with Bircher, this definition is holistic, as it includes the three major dimensions: social, physical and emotional. However, it differs from WHO and Bircher in that it emphasizes the "ability to adapt and self-manage." The main issue is that it deviates most strongly from WHO, by veering away from "complete" in terms of social, biological and mental health, rather individuals adjust to circumstances and cope according to their capacities. This is why the definition stresses that health should be viewed as "a dynamic balance between opportunities and limitations, shifting through life" (Huber et al. 2011) and affected by a number of conditions. According to this definition, those living with chronic conditions who are able to adapt and carry on with life are positively living. Huber et al. (2011) asserted that, "by successfully adapting to an illness, people are able to work or to participate in social activities and feel healthy despite limitations." So to them, "the maintenance of physiological homoeostasis" and "ability to self-manage (with a sense of coherence and fulfilled obligations) irrespective of a disease condition" are the fundamental indices of health.

But years before the definition (i.e., Huber et al.'s) was proposed, Sartorius (2006) questioned whether an ability to adapt or cope is sufficient to declare someone healthy. Sartorius (2006) observed that it is possible to have abnormal-ities (that can be counted as symptoms) without feeling sick, just as it is possible to have no abnormalities yet still feel sick. He cited examples of "people who have peptic ulcers and other diseases, experience no problems, do not know that they have a disease and do not seek treatment for it." Sartorius (2006) concluded that some of these individuals would meet both Bircher's and Huber's definitions of health because they function well for their age and within their culture yet they require medical attention. It is possible to be in an early stage of disease that could respond well to treatment; in this case, they would be identified erroneously as healthy. The definition might also be inimical to screening efforts since it is only through screening that subclinical illness be detected.

What these criticisms and counter criticisms imply is that it is difficult to have a perfect description of health. Hence, the debate might still continue as to how best to define health, which will be acceptable to all without any criticisms. The next concept is "access to health."

1.3   What does "Access to Health" Mean?

In a general sense, "access" simply means to have the opportunity to use or benefit from something. But when it comes to access to health, it is complex and multidi-mensional. It requires rigorous conceptualization, and in practical terms, it requires a lot of efforts and policies. It can be argued that creating access to health is the singular greatest problem confronting all nations in terms of healthcare. All major issues (including health system, rationing in healthcare, rights to healthcare and healthcare financing) center on access to health. The critical question in terms of wellbeing is how to ensure access to healthcare among all segments of a popu-lation, either by stressing on equality or equity. Andersen, McCutcheon, Aday, Chiu, and Bell (1983) observed that improved access to medical care has been a major goal of much health legislation and planning, and efforts to conceptualize and measure access have varied. What then is access to health?

Over three decades ago, Andersen et al. (1983) proposed two approaches to assessing/measuring access to health: (1) via population characteristics (denoted by family income, insurance coverage, attitudes toward medical care) and (2) via system characteristics (denoted by overall healthcare system, distribution and organization of manpower and facilities). In this regard, factors enabling or hinder-ing demands for healthcare are twofold: obstacles affecting supply, and population characteristics. Considering this perspective, Levesque, Harris, and Russell (2013) defined an individual's access to health as the opportunity to identify healthcare needs, to seek healthcare services, to reach, obtain or use healthcare services, and to actually have a need for services fulfilled. This individual-level approach focuses on the ability to observe health needs and to seek healthcare services. Therefore, the ease with which an individual in need of health services is able to obtain them is called "access to health."

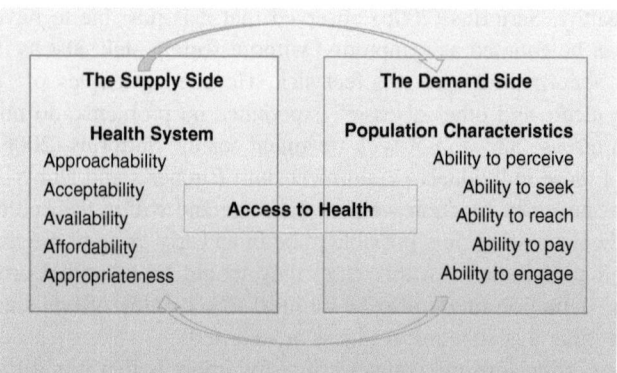

Fig. 1.1 Dimensions of access with population characteristics

In a similar vein, access to health is defined as the ability to use a service or approach a provider or an institution; thus defined as the opportunity or ease with which consumers or communities are able to use appropriate services in proportion to their needs, i.e., "opportunities to use health care facilities and obtain quality care without constraints" (Amzat & Razum, 2014, p. 77). Therefore, factors to consider include supply-side features of health systems and organizations, demand-side features of populations, and other process factors that could serve as influencers (Levesque et al. 2013). It is in line with the foregoing that Levesque et al. (2013) identified five dimensions of access to health and five abilities on the demand side (see Fig. 1.1). On the health system (supply) side, the dimensions include: approachability, acceptability, availability, affordability and appropriateness. On the population (demand) side, there are five corresponding abilities that interact with the dimensions of accessibility to generate access: ability to perceive, ability to seek, ability to reach, ability to pay, and ability to engage. The five dimensions from the side of the health system will be briefly explained.

1.3.1 Approachability

The first dimension, approachability, concerns the existence of services and the knowledge of their existence by those in need; it is not enough for services to exist if populations needing those services are unaware of their existence. The health system's contribution to approachability might involve outreach to the community in need. On the population side, this dimension corresponds to the ability to perceive need for care and to identifying where and when those services are available, based on prior information. Having such perception of need might however be dependent on the level of education, health literacy and health beliefs of the individual and the community at large. For instance, a mobile provider takes services to the people— makes efforts in reaching the community. This could be more approachable in a typical rural African village than a conventional healthcare facility. This is the same pattern in polio immunization in many African countries, following house-house strategy. This has helped in Niger and Nigeria and other countries in efforts to eradicate polio (see Curry, Perry, Tirmizi, Goldstein, & Lynch, 2014).

1.3.2   Acceptability

Even when outreach activities or mobile services are available, acceptance of those services cannot be assumed. For instance, there have been reported cases of rejection of polio vaccination in many African countries based on socio-cultural (including religious) beliefs. In some extreme cases, service providers have been harmed or even killed in northern Nigeria as a sign of rejection of vaccination (see McNeil, 2013). As observed by Levesque et al. (2013), a society forbidding casual physical contact between unmarried men and women would likely reduce acceptability of care for women if the health service providers were mostly men. The issue of gender concordance is one of the major factors affecting acceptability of maternal health services in Mali, Gambia, and other predominantly Muslim areas (Ganle, 2015). Acceptability might also be a reflection of the autonomy or personal choice of an individual to seek care. For instance, a woman who is dependent upon the decision of her husband to access care is limited in her ability to seek care. Generally, in the African setting, acceptability is moderated by certain socio-cultural and religious norms. Because of this, it is, vital that information, explanations, and treatments take social values and local concepts of illness into account (Obrist et al. 2007). Healthcare-providers must be culturally sensitive, consider local notions and systematically correct any misconceptions or misinformation. This is why even when some countries (including Ghana, Kenya, Malawi) endorse free access to some essential health services, the question of general acceptability is still paramount.

1.3.3   Availability

This mainly concerns the availability of a physical structure and qualified health personnel. The WHO recommends that healthcare facilities be available, at most, within a 5 km radius of a given population, and that reaching them does not exceed a 30-min travel time (Delamater, Messina, Shortridge, & Grady, 2012). A lack of such sufficient and functioning health facilities or qualified or trained personnel calls into question availability. Logistics issues such as location and transportation systems are also relevant here. When the road is not accessible or motorable, availability is questionable. In rural areas, many individuals or communities face the combined challenges of excessive travel time and a lack of modern transportation, which may account for a delay in health seeking. Levesque et al. (2013) averred that ability to reach healthcare is strongly linked to the notion of personal mobility, availability of transportation, occupational flexibility and knowledge about health services. The critical gap in availability of healthcare can be observed in previous and current conflict-ridden countries such as Burundi, Liberia, Eritrea, Rwanda, Somalia, Sierra Leone, and South Sudan, where the few health and associated infrastructures have been destroyed (see Guha-Sapir & D'Aoust, 2010).

1.3.4 Affordability

This primarily relates to the economic aspect of healthcare access. The critical question is "at what costs is healthcare available?" In most African countries, healthcare is still financed through fee for service (or out-of-pocket payments). As such, those who are living below the poverty-line might not be able to afford care. When healthcare is expensive, even many of those living above the poverty-line might not have the ability to pay. It is important to note that, apart from the direct costs, there are often associated costs, such as transportation fare and absenteeism from the workplace. Both direct and associated costs must be affordable. Throughout the world, financial barriers adversely affect healthcare utilization, even when services are readily available. In situations where there is a high level of poverty, access to health is particularly in jeopardy. Xu et al. (2003) have found that higher levels of out-of-pocket payments are strongly associated with exclusion from health facilities, poor response to disease symptoms and, in the long run, adversely affects household socioeconomic standing. Financial accessibility is one major factor in the debate about which healthcare system (capitalist or socialist) will promote universal care. This is why financial protection (in case of emergency, old age and related social conditions) is crucial in mitigating the financial burdens of healthcare.

1.3.5 Appropriateness

Appropriateness of healthcare addresses a number of key issues, including effectiveness of care (based on valid evidence), efficiency (cost-effectiveness), and consistency with the preferences of the relevant individual, community or society (WHO, 2000). Such healthcare should also be sustainable. Appropriateness is what Obrist et al. (2007) referred to as adequacy of care, which simply means the quality and level of services available; Is there any gap between the services provided and the needs of the client? Does the organizational setup meet the patients' expectations? Appropriateness emphasizes the content and effectiveness of the healthcare available. While some individuals require advanced care, others require only essential care according to healthcare priorities. In most African rural areas, high-tech healthcare services are not usually the main priorities. The basic and essential services such as immunization, maternal and child healthcare, family planning, and information on prevention of diseases are usually of great importance. That is why primary healthcare centres are usually sited in the rural areas to provide these essential services. In cases where advanced care is necessary, appropriate referrals are made. The technical qualities of the services provided should match the expectations and needs of the clients. Determination of adequacy of the care provided might be based on ability to engage—that is to be involved or participate in the provision of services, and on treatment decisions.

1.4   Universal Health Care (UCH)

Health-related issues constitute part of the core in the agenda of every nation. This is why how to achieve universal health care (UHC) is part of the healthcare agenda of most nations. This is for the fact that no nation is exonerated from health problems. The health status of the population is one of the elements determining the overall performance of the society. Apart from imposing financial hardships, ill-health also reduces individual capacity to function in the society. Health problems also negatively affect general economic growth. Healthcare simply means taking care of the sick or ill and prevention of such sickness or illness. Healthcare delivery by a nation is principally concerned with the delivery of preventive and curative services. Another key concept that has attracted attention in healthcare delivery systems is the notion of UHC. It is sometimes referred to as universal health coverage, universal coverage or universal care. Regardless of the terminology used, it is an overall health goal in much of the world. Although it is closely linked with access to healthcare, UHC is a distinct concept. WHO (2010) observed that the members' resolution in 2005 revived commitment to UHC—that is, to developing health financing systems so that all people have access to health services and do not suffer financial hardship paying for them. In short, UHC "means that all people can use the promotive, preventive, curative, rehabilitative and palliative health services they need, of sufficient quality to be effective, while also ensuring that the use of these services does not expose the user to financial hardship" (WHO, 2016). This is another strong bid to ensure all-inclusive access to healthcare without any form of discrimination and associated challenges (especially financial challenges). This is a global health goal as (strictly) there is no country where UHC firmly exists. The African region, however, has a longer way to go than most regions in achieving UHC. The definition of UHC includes three interrelated aspects, which will be briefly highlighted in relation to the African context.

1.4.1   Need Principle

This aspect is closely linked to socialized or socialist healthcare systems (see Sect. 3.3). It implies that the distribution and allocation of healthcare services should not be based on ability to pay but rather on need. Every individual worldwide needs some form of health services in their lifetime. While the timing and degree of need may vary, it should never be a yardstick in accessing care. In other words, healthcare should be available irrespective of individual attributes (such as income, sex, occupation, migration status). This is closely related to the right to health based on a non-discriminatory basis (see also Sect. 2.3.3). Apart from the notion of need, the services must be of sufficient quality to resolve any health need. This requires adequate and equitable distribution of good-quality healthcare infrastructures and human resources. Quality healthcare means provision of safe, accessible and efficient services in a timely manner with the best possible outcomes. Achieving this goal requires coordinated efforts and funding. While many nations, especially in the developing world, are still battling with availability and affordability, ensuring quality is for many, a tremendous challenge.

1.4.2   Financial Protection

The second component of UHC is financial protection against any health condition at any stage of life. Financial burden has been a major consequence of ill-health. The situation is particularly bad in sub-Saharan Africa (SSA), where, in the face of illness, poor families become poorer. This can be catastrophic when families must, for example, auction off their assets in order to offset healthcare bills. Because of cost, many households cannot access modern healthcare, leading some to resort to traditional medicine, more out of need than out of choice. In the absence of financial protection, health bills drain households of financial resources, which could have been used for other priorities. Globally, about 150 million people suffer financial catastrophe annually, while 100 million are pushed below poverty-line as a consequence of huge health bills (WHO, 2010, p. x). In SSA, a major problem is a heavy reliance on out-of-pocket settlement of health bills. In order to resolve this problem, there must be financial contributions covered by the government or government-supported schemes, such as pooled funds, prepayment schemes, increased government spending and international assistance (Ooms et al., 2014), ultimately resulting in the gradual elimination of direct payment by the patient and social protection covering all healthcare costs.

1.4.3   Population Coverage

The entire population of any country has the right to benefit or use all healthcare services (prevention, promotion, treatment and rehabilitation). There is no alternative to universal coverage if the right to health for all must be achieved. "Ultimately, universal coverage requires a commitment to covering 100% of the population, and plans to this end need to be developed from the outset even if the objective will not be achieved immediately" (WHO, 2010, p. xvi). Perhaps, within the Global Goals (2015–2030), every nation will move close to achieving total population coverage. This implies that every segment of the population (irrespective of personal characteristics) should have access to healthcare. If there are quality services according to need and financial protection is ensured, this automatically translates to adequate population coverage. This is the ultimate goal to be achieved in the long run. Total coverage in its true sense implies that there should not be waiting-list or criteria in accessing certain services. There should be equity in access to health services. Like when human rights are discussed, one prime feature is universality. Human rights are rights that apply to all human beings, so right to health should be universal.

1.5 Healthcare System

A healthcare system consists of all organizations, people, and actions with the primary intent to promote, restore, or maintain health (WHO, 2007, p. 2). According to WHO (2010) the aims of the health system include the following:

1. Improving the health status of individuals, families and communities.
2. Defending the population against what threatens its health.
3. Protecting people against the financial consequences of ill-health.
4. Providing equitable access to people-centered care.
5. Making it possible for people to participate in decisions affecting their health and health system.

The health system goes beyond the four walls of a hospital; it involves addressing determinants of health. WHO has long recognized that the circumstances in which people grow, reside, and work strongly influence how they live and die (CSDH, 2008). Education, socioeconomic status, housing, food and employment are all social determinants of health. Inequalities in health are reflections of the determinants of health. Health systems also include care given in the home, which is where health begins. It can range from infant nutrition to the maintenance of a first aid box in case of injury or emergency. Health systems also include various efforts at behavior change regarding dietary, sexual behavior, drug use and other lifestyles factors. Health-related legislation and policies also constitute a significant part of the health system. A health system can thus be defined as a complex structure that includes all relevant issues that can impact on population health.

WHO (2007) recognized six major building blocks of the health system, which will be briefly explained in the next few subsections. The building blocks are interwoven and interdependent to ensure the effectiveness of the health system (see Fig. 1.2).

Fig. 1.2 The six building
blocks of a health system.
Source WHO 2007:5

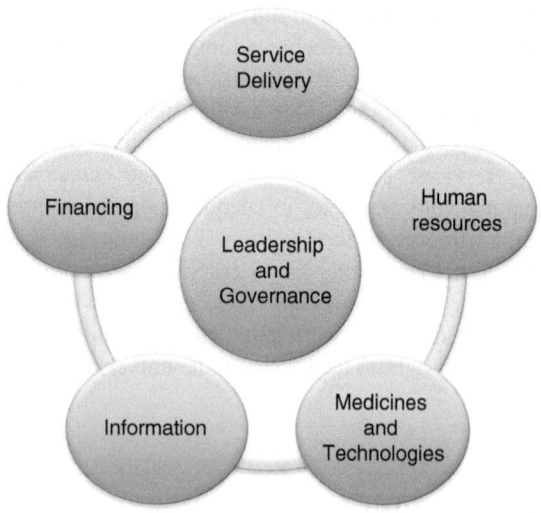

1.5.1 Health Workforce

This is represented as human resources in Fig. 1.2. It includes all cadres of staff
working towards the achievement of health goals, especially the aims of the
health system earlier specified. It starts from the lowest to the highest rank,
from those in the direct healthcare line to the auxiliaries and other associated/
allied staff. Habte, Dussault, and Dovlo (2004) described health workers as the
most important of the health system's input. According to WHO (2007), the
workforce must be sufficient in number. This has been a major challenge in
Africa, where the overall number of health workers is grossly inadequate.
Despite high disease burden, Africa produces the lowest number of basic health
workers (including community health workers, disease surveillance workers,
vaccinators, family health assistants and health information assistants). WHO
(2007) observed that extreme shortages of health workers exist in 57 countries,
36 of which are in Africa. Further compounding this shortage is the high rate of
migration of health professionals out of Africa into other parts of the world.
A 2009 report indicated that Africa has 2.3 healthcare workers per 1000 population, compared with the Americas, which have 24.8 healthcare workers per
1000 population (Naicker, Plange-Rhule, Tutt, & Eastwood, 2009). Another
concern is how to ensure fair distribution of the health workforce, as the rural
areas bear the greater brunt of the understaffing of the health workforce. Other
vital issues include training, responsiveness and productivity. There must be an
appropriate mix of various specializations, and they must be responsive to the
health needs of the population.

1.5.2 Service Delivery

The second building block is service delivery. The health system delivers an array of services including promotive, preventive, treatment and rehabilitative services to the general public. The performance is judged on the basis of effectiveness, safety, efficiency and coverage. Service delivery encompasses the home, the community and the health facility. The main concern about coverage is the proportion of the population who has access to the services. Service delivery is about quality healthcare reaching those who need it at the appropriate time. It requires the collaboration of both private and public sectors. Any gaps in service delivery, such as health service type, must be bridged. This is why comprehensive services are usually advocated. However, due to inadequate staff, many services are unavailable in many health facilities. The gap between demand and supply is a constant reality in Africa.

1.5.3 Health Information

Development and dissemination of health information is a major component of a comprehensive health system. Information regarding prevention, screening, and treatment activities is vital for empowering people to take charge of their own health and to ensure good health outcomes. Appropriate processing and thorough dissemination of health information can improve population health literacy and enhance the capacity to obtain and utilize health information to improve personal health status. Schooling ensures not only the ability to read and write, and in the long run to develop sound judgment, but it is also a major way of accessing health information. The relatively low literacy level in many African adversely affects population health. Overall, education is a determinant of health. Education affects life choices including health and illness behavior. Specifically, inadequate health information is correlated with poor health outcomes. Health information is also important for the effectiveness of health programs, especially those targeting behavior change.

1.5.4 Health Financing

Funding is central to achieving the aims of any health system; it attracts an appropriate health workforce and increases motivation and incentives for their retention and productivity, and it allows for the procurement of medical technologies as well as the construction of health facilities. Funding is also relevant to the issue of affordability raised earlier (see Sect. 1.3.4). WHO (2007) observed that each year, up to 100 million people are impoverished as a result of health spending. Healthcare systems must be financed in such a way that they are available and affordable to all and ensure financial protection to those in need of services. Although it is primarily the political sphere that is responsible for allocation and utilization of health funding (health financing is mainly assessed through government budgetary allocation for health (see also Sect. 4.2), there are other sources of finance, such as foreign aid and private sector contributions.

1.5.5 Leadership and Governance

Politics is of paramount importance in all health systems. This is because most vital decisions affecting the health system are made within the political sphere; management and allocation of resources, construction of health facilities, distribution of such facilities, employment of medical personnel, establishment of medical schools, allocation of funds for health programs, and overall policy formulation, acceptance and implementation all rest within the realm of politics. By implications, some fundamental factors affecting supply of healthcare are beyond the medical practitioners. Strong political determination is a major driving force of the overall performance of the health system. Following this, WHO (2007, p. iv) observed that leadership and governance in the health system "involves ensuring strategic policy frameworks exist and are combined with effective oversight, coalition-building, regulation, attention to system-design and accountability." In addition, apart from the overall political framework at the macro level, there is also micro level governance within the health sector. The technical inputs, coordination and service delivery also require appropriate organizational/leadership structure, without which services might not be appropriately supplied.

1.5.6 Medical Products, Vaccines and Technologies

The final building block has to do with essential medicines and equipment. Essential medical products, vaccines and technologies must be available in appropriate quantity and quality. A fundamental assertion is that in most developing countries, essential medicine is available more often in the private sector than in the public sector (WHO, 2007, p. 9). It is further observed that "an estimated 50% of medical equipment in developing countries is not used, either because of a lack of spare parts or maintenance, or because health workers do not know how to use it." Finally, and of vital importance, an infrequent and irregular power supply keeps health personnel from putting any existing equipment to use.

References

Amzat, J., & Razum, O. (2014). *Medical sociology in Africa*. Cham, Switzerland: Springer International Publishing.

Andersen, R. M., McCutcheon, A., Aday, L. A., Chiu, G. Y., Bell, R. (1983). Exploring dimensions of access to medical care. *Health Services Research, 18*(1), 49–74.

Bircher, J. (2005). Towards a dynamic definition of health and disease. *Medicine, Health Care and Philosophy, 8*, 335–341.

CSDH (2008). *Closing the gap in a generation: health equity through action on the social determinants of health. Final Report of the Commission on Social Determinants of Health*. Geneva: World Health Organization.

Curry, D. W., Perry, H. B., Tirmizi, S. N., Goldstein, A. L., Lynch, M. C. (2014). Assessing the effectiveness of house-to-house visits on routine oral polio immunization completion and tracking of defaulters. *Journal of Health, Population and Nutrition, 32*(2), 356–366.

Delamater, P. L., Messina, J. P., Shortridge, A. M., Grady, S. C. (2012). Measuring geographic access to health care: raster and network-based methods. *International Journal of Health Geographics, 11*, 15. doi:10.1186/1476-072X-11-15.

Ganle, J. K. (2015). Why Muslim women in Northern Ghana do not use skilled maternal healthcare services at health facilities: a qualitative study. *BMC International Health and Human Rights, 15*(1), 10. doi:10.1186/s12914-015-0048-9.

Godlee, F. (2011). What is health? *British Medical Journal, 343*, d4817.

Guha-Sapir, D., & D'Aoust, O. (2010). Demographic and health consequences of civil conflict. World Development Report 2011 Background Paper.

Habte, D., Dussault, G., Dovlo, D. (2004). Challenges confronting the health workforce in sub-Saharan Africa. *World Hospitals and Health Services: the Official Journal of the International Hospital Federation, 40*(2), 23–26. 40–41.

Huber, M., Knottnerus, J. A., Green, L., van der Horst, H., Jadad, A. R., Kromhout, D., et al. (2011). How should we define health? *British Medical Journal, 343*, d4163. doi:10.1136/bmj.d4163.

Jadad, A. R., & O'Grady, L. (2008). How should health be defined? *British Medical Journal, 337*, a2900. doi:10.1136/bmj.a2900.

Levesque, J., Harris, M. F., Russell, G. (2013). Patient-centred access to health care: conceptualising access at the interface of health systems and populations. *International Journal for Equity in Health, 12*, 18.

McNeil, D. G. (2013, February 8). Gunmen kill Nigerian polio vaccine workers in echo of Pakistan attacks. *The New York Times*. http://www.nytimes.com/2013/02/09/world/africa/in-nigeria-polio-vaccine-workers-are-killed-by-gunmen.html. Accessed July 7, 2017.

Naicker, S., Plange-Rhule, J., Tutt, R. C., Eastwood, J. B. (2009). Shortage of healthcare workers in developing countries: Africa. *Ethnicity & Disease, 19*(1 Suppl 1), S1-60–S1-64.

Obrist, B., Iteba, N., Lengeler, C., Makemba, A., Mshana, C., Nathan, R., et al. (2007). Access to health care in contexts of livelihood insecurity: a framework for analysis and action. *PLoS Medicine, 4*(10), e308. doi:10.1371/journal.pmed.0040308.

Ooms, G., Latif, L. A., Waris, A., Brolan, C. E., Hammonds, R., Friedman, E. A., et al. (2014). Is universal health coverage the practical expression of the right to health care? *BMC International Health and Human Rights, 14*, 3.

Parsons, T. (1972). Definition of health and illness in the light of American values and social structure. In E. G. Jaco (Ed.). *Patients, physicians and illness* (pp. 107–127). New York: Free Press.

Saracci, R. (1997). The World Health Organization needs to reconsider its definition of health. *British Medical Journal, 314*, 1409–1410.

Sartorius, N. (2006). The meanings of health and its promotion. *Croatian Medical Journal, 47*, 662–664.

Simmons, A. M. (1998, September 30). Where fat is a mark of beauty. *Los Angeles Times*, p. 23–24.

Üstün, B., & Jakob, R. (2005). Calling a spade a spade: meaningful definitions of health conditions. *Bulletin of the World Health Organization, 83*, 802.

WHO (1946). Preamble to the Constitution of the World Health Organization as adopted by the International Health Conference, New York, 19–22 June, 1946.

WHO (2000). Appropriateness in Health Care Services. Report on a WHO Workshop, Koblenz, Germany, 23–25 March 2000.

WHO (2007). *Everybody's business: strengthening health systems to improve health outcomes: WHO's framework for action.* Geneva: WHO.

WHO (2010). *The World Health Report: health systems financing: the path to universal coverage.* Geneva: WHO.

WHO (2016). *Health Financing for Universal Coverage.* http://www.who.int/health_financing/universal_coverage_definition/en/. Accessed May 17 2016.

Xu, K., Evans, D. B., Kawabata, K., Zeramdini, R., Klavus, J., Murray, C. J. L. (2003). Household catastrophic health expenditure: a multicountry analysis. *Lancet, 362*, 111–117.

Chapter 2
The Right to Health in Africa

2.1 Introduction

This chapter focuses on the concept of the right to healthcare. In general, the right to health is an ambitious yet unfulfilled promise to humanity in many parts of the world. This includes Africa, the continent with the highest burden of most diseases, especially preventable diseases, including malaria, TB and HIV/AIDS. The continent is locked in a vulnerability complex made manifest in and through underdevelopment, global health inequalities and health system failures, including poor healthcare delivery. This all combines to ensure that the disease burden in Africa remains very high, and why the right to healthcare in the region is still a mirage.

Regardless of age, gender, socio-economic or ethnic background, health is humanity's most basic and essential asset (WHO, 2016), which facilitate functional roles in the society (i.e., participation in community activities). This is why the right to health should not be negotiable but guaranteed unconditionally. The right to health is actually, in its full sense, the "right of everyone to the enjoyment of the highest attainable standard of physical and mental health," often shortened to the "right to the highest attainable standard of health" or simply, the "right to health" (see Hunt, 2006; Box 2.1). It is believed that if the right to health is guaranteed, the world will be a better place for all in terms of access to quality healthcare or universal healthcare. Granting the right to health has been one of the reasons behind most health campaigns meant to ensure population coverage of healthcare. While all nations have not been able to guaranteed this right, some nations (especially the developing world) are not faring well at all. In developing countries, every right is perpetually jeopardized because of the state of socio-economic development and political issues.

© Springer International Publishing AG 2018

J. Amzat, O. Razum, *Towards a Sociology of Health Discourse in Africa*,
DOI 10.1007/978-3-319-61672-8_2

Box 2.1 The Universal Declaration of Human Rights (abbreviated)

Article 1	Right to Equality
Article 2	Freedom from Discrimination
Article 3	Right to Life, Liberty, Personal Security
Article 4	Freedom from Slavery
Article 5	Freedom from Torture and Degrading Treatment
Article 6	Right to Recognition as a Person before the Law
Article 7	Right to Equality before the Law
Article 8	Right to Remedy by Competent Tribunal
Article 9	Freedom from Arbitrary Arrest and Exile
Article 10	Right to Fair Public Hearing
Article 11	Right to be Considered Innocent until Proven Guilty
Article 12	Freedom from Interference with Privacy, Family, Home and Correspondence
Article 13	Right to Free Movement in and out of the Country
Article 14	Right to Asylum in other Countries from Persecution
Article 15	Right to a Nationality and the Freedom to Change It
Article 16	Right to Marriage and Family
Article 17	Right to Own Property
Article 18	Freedom of Belief and Religion
Article 19	Freedom of Opinion and Information
Article 20	Right of Peaceful Assembly and Association
Article 21	Right to Participate in Government and in Free Elections
Article 22	Right to Social Security
Article 23	Right to Desirable Work and to Join Trade Unions
Article 24	Right to Rest and Leisure
Article 25	Right to Adequate Living Standard [Adequate for Health]
Article 26	Right to Education
Article 27	Right to Participate in the Cultural Life of Community
Article 28	Right to a Social Order that Articulates this Document
Article 29	Community Duties Essential to Free and Full Development
Article 30	Freedom from State or Personal Interference in the above Rights

Source Flowers (1999).

Irrespective of the state of the right to health across different regions, efforts for its fulfilment would definitely continue because it is fundamental aspect of human dignity. Right to health is important because:

1. Right to health signifies a global and national commitment through a legal framework. This is why there have been a number of international documents reaffirming the legal basis of the right, which many nations have signed and made part of their domestic policies. This domestication is important for the law to take effect or be implemented for the benefits of all.

2. Constitutional provision for the right to health often serves as a guiding principle for domestic policies and international relations. Such provision will shape domestic policies by enforcing (to some extent) practical commitment in meeting the expectations.
3. It specifies specific rights to individuals under any jurisdiction. Some of those rights are connected with other rights and human right principles. For instance, the right to health is linked to the right to water and other social amenities. It is not just about healthcare, but also specific infrastructures that can enhance better health condition.
4. It is about the state obligations corresponding with those rights—obligation to respect, protect and fulfil the rights of every individual. Specifically, most of the international treaties on right to health highlight what need to be done for the fulfilment of the right. The rules create direction towards the realization of the right.
5. It is also about mechanisms to monitor states' compliance with their obligations and allows individuals to seek redress for violations of their rights. If a constitutional right is violated, it is possible to seek redress. This can invariably motivate the government to meet such expectations.

Having highlighted the importance of "right to health," the rest of the chapter will focus on the conceptual issues such as right to health and human right principles relevant to health, and the relationship between human rights and health.

2.2 International Documents and the Right to Health

The right to the enjoyment of the highest attainable standard of physical and mental health, was first articulated in the 1946 Constitution of the World Health Organization, which stated that the right to health is one of the fundamental rights of every human being irrespective of race, religion, political belief, economic or social condition (WHO, 1948; WHO, 2016). Other provisions, of particular relevance to Africa, include:

1. Universal Declaration of Human Rights (Article 25)
2. International Covenant on Economic, Social and Cultural Rights (Article 12)
3. African Charter on Human and Peoples' Rights (Article 16)

In 1948, the United Nations (UN) affirmed the right to health in Article 25 of its Universal Declaration of Human Rights, that "Everyone has the right to a standard of living adequate for the health and well-being of himself and of his family, including food, clothing, housing and medical care and necessary social services, and the right to security in the event of unemployment, sickness, disability, widowhood, old age or other lack of livelihood in circumstances beyond his control. [And that] Motherhood and childhood are entitled to special care and assistance. All children, whether born in or out of wedlock, shall enjoy the same social protection." The Declaration is highly explicit, it also acknowledges the right to health in the context of one of the determinants of health, "(an adequate) standard of living," while also including medical care and security in the event of sickness as basic rights (see Box 2.1 for the abbreviated list of human rights).

The International Covenant on Economic, Social and Cultural Rights (ICESCR), adopted in 1966 and entered into force on January 3, 1976, also recognizes the right to health. Article 12 of the ICESCR, states that parties must recognize "the right of everyone to the enjoyment of the highest attainable standard of physical and mental health." The article spells out some practical steps "to achieve the full realization of this right," including:

1. The provision for the reduction of the stillbirth-rate and of infant mortality and for the healthy development of the child;
2. The improvement of all aspects of environmental and industrial hygiene;
3. The prevention, treatment and control of epidemic, endemic, occupational and other diseases;
4. The creation of conditions, which would assure to all (individuals) medical service and medical attention in the event of sickness.

Universal recognition of the right to health was further confirmed in the 1978 Declaration of Alma-Ata on Primary Healthcare, with the vision of "health for all" by the year 2000 (WHO, 1978). This led to the introduction of PHC in most African countries to provide sustainable and basic healthcare to all. Nearly all African countries are also signatories to the UN, and to the other major human rights documents. This includes the African Charter on Human and Peoples' Rights (also known as the Banjul Charter) (adopted in 1981), which is intended to promote and protect human rights and basic freedoms throughout the African continent. Article 16 (1 and 2) is specifically titled "Right to Health" and states that "Every individual shall have the right to enjoy the best attainable state of physical and mental health. State Parties to the present Charter shall take the necessary measures to protect the health of their people and to ensure that they receive medical attention when they are sick." This recognizes the responsibility of every state to provide healthcare services to all individuals, without exception. The right to health is further expanded upon in the 2011 Guidelines and Principles on Economic, Social and Cultural Rights in the African Charter on Human and Peoples' Rights as follows:

1. The right to health is an inclusive right that encompasses both healthcare and the underlying determinants of health. The right to health does not mean the right to be healthy because being healthy is a function of numerous pre-determined conditions (including physiological conditions).
2. The right to healthcare requires an effective and integrated health system, which is responsive to national and local priorities, and accessible to all.
3. The determinants of health include access to safe and potable water and adequate sanitation, an adequate supply of safe food, nutrition and housing, healthy occupational and environmental conditions.
4. The right to health includes effective access to health-related education and information, including on sexual and reproductive health. It also includes

freedoms such as control over one's own body and health, including sexual and reproductive freedom.

5. The individual has the right to be free from unwarranted interference, including non-consensual medical treatment, experimentation, forced sterilization and inhuman and degrading treatment.

While the Banjul Charter and further codification have been laudable, achieving the set rules has been very slow. The main challenge to realizing the aims has been about incorporating the articles into domestic policy and practical implementation. The "health for all by the year 2000" could not be achieved in many parts of the world. The same can be said for the health aspects of the Millennium Development Goals (MDGs), which were not (totally) achieved by 2015, especially in SSA and other parts of the developing world. Currently, there are Sustainable Development Goals (SDGs) (also known as Global Goals) meant to be achieved by 2030.

A number of African countries have taken further steps, through constitutional provisions, to recognize and integrate the right to health into their domestic policies. A 2010 report reviewed constitutional provisions on the right to health in 14 countries in east and southern Africa (ESA), including Angola, Botswana, Kenya, Lesotho, Madagascar, Malawi, Mozambique, Namibia, South Africa, Swaziland, Tanzania, Uganda, Zimbabwe and Zambia, plus Congo Brazzaville (Mulumba, Kabanda, & Nassuna, 2010). The report drew connections between access to health and the minimum essential food, basic shelter and sanitation, essential drugs to right to healthcare. They observed that, although many constitutions expressly provide for the right to health, in others this right can only be inferred indirectly from other rights. The report indicated a number of "best practices" in constitutional provisions:

1. Mozambique's constitution provides for the right of access to health facilities, goods and services on a non-discriminatory basis.
2. Uganda's constitution provides provisions for access to food that is nutritionally adequate and safe, and ensures freedom from hunger for everyone.
3. South Africa's constitution makes provisions for access to basic shelter, housing and sanitation, and an adequate supply of safe and potable water. The constitution also provides for healthcare, food, water and social security.
4. Malawi's constitution is also a good reference point regarding the national public health strategy addressing the health concerns of the whole population. The Constitution recognizes provision of adequate nutrition for all in order to promote good health and self-sufficiency, and provision of adequate healthcare, commensurate with the health needs of Malawian society and international standards of healthcare.

In general, South Africa is a good reference point when discussing constitutional provision of the right to health in Africa (Pieterse, 2014). It explicitly states, in Constitution Chapter II, Section 27 that: "everyone has the right to have access to healthcare services, including reproductive healthcare sufficient food and water;

[…] and 2. the State must take reasonable legislative and other measures, within its available resources, to achieve the progressive realization of each of these rights; and (3) No one may be refused emergency medical treatment." Efforts are gradually being made to fully realize the constitutional provisions. As previously observed, majority of African States are signatories to documents about the right to health. However, the problem is often about domestication and implementation.

2.3   Human Rights Principles Relevant To Health Issues

Human rights, as per international law, are rights that every human being possesses, irrespective of individual attributes, such as race/ethnicity, religious or political beliefs, legal status, economic status, gender, language, color and nationality. The rights are fundamental to human essence such as human dignity and integrity. Violation of such rights constitutes defilement of humanity and should be disapproved in all ramifications. One critical question surrounding the right to health is whether it should be conceptualized as a human right. Are there links between health and other human rights, such as right to life and education? The general notion is that challenges to human rights constitute a threat to the basis of humanity—to human general wellbeing (Amzat, 2015). It is further explained that a rights-based consideration upholds the centrality of the human person, with a compelling reference to the fundamental human rights of every person (Amzat, 2015).

Rights discourse is fundamentally linked to health issues considering the principles or dimensions of human rights. It is impossible to guarantee healthcare without protection and fulfillment of human rights. The principles underlying human rights hold fundamental implications for health indicators of the population. This is why human rights documents advocate the right to health as a basic human right with entitlement and obligations including some practical measures in realizing health for all. It is on this note that Leary (1994) identified a number of dimensions/principles of human rights, which are relevant to the conceptualization of health as human rights. The principles will be briefly discussed.

2.3.1   Human Rights as a Social or Public Goal

The crucial point is that the use of rights language in connection with health issues elevates the importance of healthcare and health status (Leary, 1994). Rights are crucial to the basis of statehood in connection to the citizenry. Rights are essential ingredients of any nation. The same applies to healthcare; it is an important basis of any nation. Rights and healthcare reflect in socio-political wellbeing. There is a strong association between health indicators and level of socio-economic development. When health indicators (including mortality, morbidity, disability, healthcare utilization rates) are bad, the level of productivity and development in a country will generally be low. Therefore, "conceptualizing health status in terms of rights under-scores health as a social good and not solely a medical, technical, or economic problem" (Leary, 1994, p. 36). This also underscores the instrumentality of health in the day-day activities of the society. Health helps in the fulfillment of social roles of individuals; it is therefore instrumental to the functionality of human society in all ramifications. A social good is a common good that constitutes an essential need of everyone; an indispensable need, which everyone must access for survival. Healthcare then occupies a similar position with clean water, clean air and education. The attainment of high standards of health is a fundamental goal of every nation; so attainment of health is also a socio-public goal.

2.3.2   The Dignity of Human Person

The rights-based approach focuses on respect for human dignity, which refers to the capacity of being human with infinite value, without undue limitations in all spheres of life, which must be honored and respected (Rendtorff, 2002). Human rights are inherent, inalienable, priceless and precious. Human dignity is inviolable and must be respected and protected as its absence or violation signifies degradation and depersonalization. The dignity of the human person is not only a fundamental right in itself, but constitutes the basis of fundamental rights. This is because it signifies the "worthiness" of humanness. The same status quality is accorded to human health because it is related to human value. Another usage is that human dignity must be respected in all aspects of healthcare including medical experimentation, medical surveillance and procedures (Leary, 1994). The focus must be on the dignity of the individual rather than the good of the collectivity. The principle of human dignity rejects the objectification and instrumentation of human in healthcare and biomedicine in general. It signifies that every individual is a subject whose right must not be compromised in the name of scientific endeavor.

2.3.3   The Principle of Equality and Non-discrimination

One major aspect of the declaration of human rights is the concept of equality. Everyone is equal before the law, and rights should be guaranteed without any form of discrimination. This implies that rights should be guaranteed irrespective of personal attributes such as class, sex, race, gender and migration status or achieved status. In reality, individual characteristics (sex, race, religion, age, disability, sexual orientation and health condition [such as people living with HIV]) have been the basis for some form of discrimination in healthcare. Every nation should therefore promote social inclusion and equal opportunities for all regarding access to healthcare services and other essential needs. The notion of equality also extends to the determinants of health such as access to food, education, housing, water and sanitation. Individuals should have equal access to these essential needs, which have consequences for health status.

The South African Constitution (Section 27) contains an equality-threshold that forbids group-based distinctions in the provision of health services, and forbids arbitrary or unfair exclusion from health-related programs and provision of healthcare services (Pieterse, 2014). Beyond constitutional provisions, every nation must critically review all types of barriers to equal access to healthcare. It is important that discrimination is challenged and services are adapted to the needs of vulnerable groups who are likely to suffer from discrimination. For instance, even the physical structure of a facility might not cater for the needs of those living with disability, and therefore systematically prevent them from accessing health facilities. The bottom-line is that in healthcare, every life should be of equal value to another.

2.3.4 The Principle of Public Participation

Individuals should be properly engaged in the planning and implementation of health programs. This will generate a sense of belonging and ownership devoid of imposition. Participation helps in agenda-setting and prioritization. In general, "public involvement refers to the involvement of members of the public in strategic decisions about health services and policy at local or national level—for instance, about the configuration of services or setting priorities" (Florin, 2004), and general healthcare policies. It is generally assumed that public involvement is necessary because public services are paid for by the people and therefore should be shaped more extensively by them to ensure accountability and transparency and democratic decision making, which will enhance efficiency and acceptability (Florin, 2004). Apart from democratizing healthcare, public participation also helps to focus on the interest of the individuals in order to ensure that the best quality of care is delivered (Staniszewska, Herron-Marx, & Mockford, 2008). In short, public participation is a major means of enhancing the responsiveness of healthcare systems. In sum, "all individuals and communities are entitled to active and informed participation on issues relating to their health. In the context of health systems, this includes participation in identifying overall strategy, policy-making, implementation and accountability" (Hunt & Backman, 2008).

2.3.5 Entitlements and Obligations

It is also important to note that rights confer some entitlements (mostly in term of provisions or programs). For instance, government can institute programs meant to meet the health needs of the individuals. An entitlement is accorded to the right holder to access to some benefits (which could be group-specific) and based on established rights or by legislation. Human rights are seen as entitlements of persons or individuals to essential goods, of which can confer some claims (Azevedo, 2010). In right discourse, identification of claims (i.e., health-related demands considered as one's due) by the right holder is important. Apart from the right holder, is the duty bearer with the obligation to provide certain entitlements. This implies that protection of right to health relies on states as the guarantor (or duty bearer) (Kingston, Cohen, & Morley, 2010). This also confers some opportunities to seek redress in the case of rights' violations. There have been a number of cases of litigation meant to enforce the right to healthcare across the world. In South Africa, for example, the AIDS advocacy group, the Treatment Action Campaign (TAC), took legal action against the government to expand the scope of HIV treatment to pregnant women based on the child's right to health (see Singh, Govender, & Mills, 2007). Some of the obligations, which the right holder is entitled to, have been identified in various international rights document such as that of the ICESCR. The obligations include ensuring the right of access to health facilities, goods and services on a non-discriminatory basis, especially for vulnerable or marginalized groups; ensuring access to the minimum essential food which is nutritionally adequate and safe; ensuring freedom from hunger; ensuring access to basic shelter, housing and sanitation, and an adequate supply of safe and potable water; providing essential drugs; ensuring equitable distribution of all health facilities, goods and services; adopting and implementing a national public health strategy and plan of action on the basis of epidemiological evidence; and addressing the health concerns of the whole population.

2.3.6   Interdependence of Rights

Rights do not exist in a vacuum—rights are interdependent and interrelated. Fulfillment of one right might be directly or indirectly connected with another right. It also means that when one right is fulfilled, the other right is positively affected. Invariably, rights are collectively considered interdependent and indivisible. It has been suggested that there is a "mutually reinforcing dynamic between different categories of rights in the sense that the effective implementation of one category of rights can contribute to the effective implementation of other categories of rights and vice versa" (Quane, 2012, p. 49). In addition, there is no hierarchy of rights; every right is of equal importance to the other.

The violation of one right also has multiplier effects on other rights. This implies that the right to health cannot be effectively protected without respect for other recognized rights including prohibition of discrimination, and the right of persons to participate in decisions affecting them (Leary, 1994). The right to education, food, good shelter, potable water, sanitation and other essential needs are closely linked with the right to health. The right to life is closely linked to the right to healthcare. For instance, if there is no quality and affordable healthcare, the life expectancy will be very low.

2.3.7 *Limitations on Rights*

Rights are not absolute. Rights sometimes might be limited because of collective interests. The right to freedom of expression has libel and slander as limits. An individual rights or entitlement should not constitute a threat to others. The right to movement might be restricted during emergencies. The same applies to the right to health as there could be limitations in certain respects when it is absolutely indispensible. A number of scholars have explained some restrictions to right to health (see Loefler, 1999; Lamm, 1998). It is often assumed that the duty bearer (the government) has unlimited resources to provide health needs for all (Loefler, 1999). Such assumption is erroneous, as it can be observed in many developing countries, the resources (both human and material) and logistics required to provide right to health are grossly inadequate. It might not be practicable to make claims in many socio-economic and political circumstances. In another dimension, for certain public health measures, right might be curtailed. It is only important that such limitation only applies when it is absolutely necessary. For instance, during Ebola crisis in Guinea, Liberia and Sierra Leone freedom of movement was largely checked in some affected quarters. Many individuals with suspected cases of Ebola were also quarantined. In this sense, for public health purpose and to protect the right to life of others in the face of epidemics, the duty bearer (the government) can impose some restrictions, which are justifiable on health grounds.

2.4 Linkages Between Human Rights and Health

There are specific human rights considerations that are closely linked to health. Hence, WHO affirmed that promoting and protecting health and respecting and fulfilling human right are inextricably linked. This is because certain practices, policies and violations can lead to ill-health in human society. Long ago Mann et al. (1994) summarized the linkages under three major frameworks (same as WHO), including human rights violations, health policies and vulnerability reduction through human rights.

2.4.1 *Health Impacts Resulting from Violations of Human Rights*

Human rights are meant to be respected and fulfilled at all times. As shown in Fig. 2.1, violations of rights often result in ill-health. Such violations might take different forms, including harmful traditional practices, torture, inhuman treatment, discrimination, slavery, and violence against women. Mann et al. (1994) observed that health impacts associated with violations of rights and dignity constitute

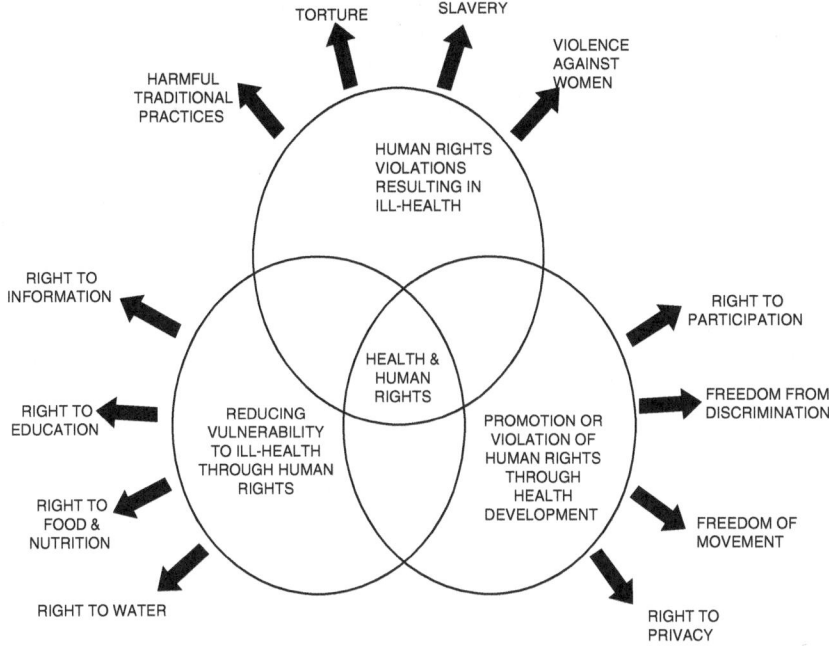

Fig. 2.1   Health and human rights linkages. *Source* WHO (2016)

significant health issues, which must be addressed. For instance, there are a number of harmful traditional practices in Africa, which constitute infraction on human rights, and adversely affect human health. Some harmful traditional practices are still thriving, including female genital cutting, forced feeding of adolescent girls, early marriage and son preference. Heise, Germain, and Pitanguy (1994) reported that there is still a high incidence of sex selection leading to abortion of the female fetus or infanticide of infant girls. Battering during pregnancy and rape are also prevalent, and in some cases are culturally sanctioned (Heise et al., 1994). Such harmful practices constitute human rights infractions and contribute to the health burden. There is also mortality inequality due to gender inequality in several countries including Angola, Chad, Somalia, Mali, Democratic Republic of the Congo, Nigeria, Sierra Leone, Guinea-Bissau, the Central African Republic, Burkina Faso, Niger, Burundi, and North African countries (Sen, 2003; World Bank, 2011). Such mortality is due to (gender-based) selective care and harmful practices.

Harmful practices (such as unnecessary scarification [facial scarification] and female genital cutting) are also human rights transgressions that can have severe health consequences. There are physical, psychological and social pains associated with female genital cutting. Also in many countries (especially in the middle East, Asia and Africa) forced marriage of young girls as low as 8 years old is still prevalent. Child marriage is often done in line with some religious and cultural expectations (e.g., based on cultural value placed upon virginity). Child marriage robs young girls of their childhood, education and future aspirations. Maternal morbidity and mortality are inextricably linked to too-early childbearing (especially before the age of 18). All human rights documents forbid harmful practice against any group of the society. For instance, harmful practices are referred to in the Convention on the Rights of the Child (Article 24(3)), Convention on the Elimination of All Forms of Discrimination against Women (CEDAW) (Articles 2, 5 and 16) and other regional instruments, drawing the attention of member states to address them.

Other critical issues include the use of torture and forced incarceration, including slavery and harsh labor practices—all of which constitute inhuman treatment/ conditions. Human rights violations hold serious adverse consequences for human health. For instance, toiling in unrewarding, unsafe and hazardous working conditions puts millions of people at health risks worldwide. Mann et al. (1994, p. 19) urged appreciation of the link between health and human rights, writing that "documentation of health impacts of rights violations may contribute to increased societal awareness of the importance of human rights promotion and protection."

2.4.2   The Impact of Health Policies, Programs and Practices on Human Rights

In general, that health policies and programs can promote or violate human rights. The state is (in most countries) in charge of who gets what and where in terms of healthcare distribution. Such allocation must be based on equitable principles and policies. This is why "right to health" and "justice in care" have been central in healthcare discourse over the years. The argument is that healthcare must be equitably distributed to all segments of the society. This means that access to healthcare must be ensured by the state (see the dimensions of access to care in Chap. 1) without discrimination. A situation where certain segment of the society is under-served because of location (especially rural areas), political or religious beliefs, is indeed against the human rights declarations. Inadequate or lack of health facilities has been widely reported in many African communities. Such deprivation is against the UDHR and Banjul Charter, and hold serious adverse health implications for such communities.

Furthermore, assessing the goals of public health (including assessing health needs and problems; developing policies designed to address priority health issues; and assuring programs to implement strategic health goals), Mann et al. (1994) observed that potential benefits to and burdens on human rights might occur while pursuing each of these major areas of public health responsibility. Mann et al. (1994) observed that through implementation of programs, right violations might occur through a number of ways. Such ways include by neglecting health circumstances of certain groups (especially the marginalized or stigmatized group); excluding certain group from health assessment and not protecting the rights of the vulnerable; and not respecting research ethics (such as principles of informed consent and non-maleficence) in pursuance of health goals. This is why research ethics signify that no group should be exempted from research activities without strong scientifically justifiable reasons.

The health program must also take the determinants of health into account. The UDHR stresses the "living condition adequate for health." When a State does not address such determinants of health (such as poverty, housing and working condition), it may amount to discrimination, which is inimical to human rights. The implication is that disease burden will be unevenly distributed and access to care might be a mirage for certain groups. The same applies to right to participation and information. As previously observed, individuals have the right to participate in issues affecting their health. Access to information (especially health information) is also critical. Many states in Africa and Middle East deprive their citizen of sexuality education, which is part of the reasons for the poor awareness and implementation of sexual and reproductive rights in the region. In design and implementation of health program including public health, respect for right principles should not be compromised arbitrarily. To do otherwise requires adequate scientific and ethical grounds.

2.4.3   Vulnerability Reduction Through Human Rights

It has also been argued that if a State takes steps to sanction human rights, vulnerability to ill-health can be reduced. As previously observed, there are many specific human rights (see Box 2.1), which are interrelated and interdependent. Population health is also determined by how the rights of individuals are respected in the society. For instance, education is a major determinant of health. If the right to education is fulfilled, it will positively affect the health indicator of a society. For instance, a study found that additional years of secondary schooling had a large protective effect against HIV risk in Botswana, particularly for women (De Neve, Fink, Subramanian, Moyo, & Bor, 2015). Schooling also helps to reduce teenage pregnancy. Karlsen et al. (2011) found that women with no education had twice the risk of maternal mortality compared to women with some education in Africa, Asia and Latin America. Apart from education, the right to food, housing and freedom from discrimination can also greatly reduce vulnerability to diseases.

2.5   Relevance of Rights Discourse to a Specific Disease: The Case of HIV

The essence of this section is to further explain how rights discourse is applicable to HIV. Particularly, how rights can be safeguarded to control vulnerability to HIV? In general, HIV raises many human rights issues, thus making protecting and promoting human rights essential for preventing the transmission of HIV and reducing the global impact of AIDS (WHO, 2016).

Historically, there have been a number of grievous concerns regarding People Living with HIV/AIDS (PLWHA), including mandatory HIV testing, restrictions on international travel, barriers to employment and housing, access to education, medical care, and/or health insurance, and partner notification and confidentiality (Gruskin & Tarantola, 2002). The relationship between HIV/AIDS and human rights is most often illustrated through the impact on the lives of the individuals infected, including neglect, denial, and violation of their rights, especially among women, children and other vulnerable groups (Gruskin & Tarantola, 2002). Some fundamental human rights such as the right to life, equality before the law, the right to privacy and the right to the highest attainable standard of health are particularly applicable. There is no better best practice than to respect, protect and fulfill these rights (see Table 2.1). The next subsections will examine some vital areas of rights-based challenges in the context of HIV/AIDS.

Table 2.1 Governmental obligations with respect to people in the context of HIV/AIDS

	People infected with HIV	People affected by HIV/AIDS	People vulnerable to HIV/AIDS
Respect	Government to refrain from directly violating the human rights of people living with HIV/AIDS on the basis of their HIV status.	Government to refrain from directly violating the rights of people affected by the HIV/AIDS pandemic.	Government to refrain from directly violating human rights that increase vulnerability.
Protect	Government is responsible for preventing rights violations by nonstate actors against people living with HIV/AIDS and for providing some legal means of redress.	Government is responsible for preventing violations by nonstate actors that would increase the burden of HIV/AIDS on affected people, and for providing some legal means of redress.	Government is responsible for preventing rights violations by nonstate actors that may increase people's vulnerability to HIV/AIDS, and for providing some legal means of redress.
Fulfill	Government to take administrative, judicial, and other measures toward realization of the rights of people living with HIV/AIDS.	Government to take administrative, legislative, judicial, and other measures toward the realization of the rights of people affected by HIV/AIDS.	Government to take administrative, legislative, judicial, and other measures toward the realization of the rights of people to minimize their vulnerability to HIV/AIDS.

Source Gruskin and Tarantola (2002).

2.5.1 Ensuring Gender Equality

In SSA, the incidence of HIV is higher among women and those living in poverty. This is due, in part, to gender discrimination and inequality. Women are technically and culturally discriminated against in terms of education, paid employment and access to asset (e.g., inheritance). Women are also poorer because they are mostly housewives and therefore financially dependent on their husbands. Some women could not complete their education, also due to gender inequality. Women are generally exposed to multiple vulnerability issues. They are also exposed to sexual assaults such as marital rape and forced marriage. Women's autonomy is generally poor (Amzat, 2015) and they suffer inhuman degradation of imposition of decision without choices. Respect for women's rights and improving their access to basic amenities of life would definitely help in reducing their vulnerability to HIV.

2.5.2 Harmful Practices as Infraction on Human Rights

The control of harmful traditional practices, which are inimical to human rights, will protect certain group against HIV/AIDS. Most of those harmful practices constitute infringement on human rights (as previous mentioned). Practices such as cleansing rituals, female genital mutilation, wife inheritance and virginity testing are clear infringement on human rights and make people vulnerable to HIV. While addressing them require some careful steps and cultural sensitivity (Maleche & Day, 2011), it is important to curtail traditional norms that are not compatible with human rights.

2.5.3 Stigma and Discrimination Inimical to Human Rights

HIV is highly associated with stigma and discrimination. UNAIDS (2014, p. 2) defined HIV-related stigma "as negative beliefs, feelings and attitude towards people living with HIV, groups associated with people living with HIV and other key populations at higher risk of HIV infection," while HIV-related discrimination refers to unfair and unjust treatment (through act or omission) of an individual based on his/her real or perceived HIV status. UNAIDS (2014) further observed that stigma and discrimination are among the foremost barriers to HIV prevention, treatment, care and support. This is because stigmatization undermines HIV prevention efforts by making people afraid to seek HIV information, services, treatment and modalities to reduce their risk of infection and to adopt safer measures of HIV prevention. Stigmatization also imposes psychological and social frustration on those living with HIV, which also makes them susceptible to various complications including untimely death. Also, HIV-related sigma is correlated to poor quality of life, poor health status, denied access to care and shame around accessed care.

2.5.4   Ensuring Access to Treatment

Universal access to care and treatment is also an important component of the right to health for persons living with HIV/AIDS (PLWHA). There is still a wide gap in HIV treatment in Africa, with 59%, 79% and 89% in East and Southern Africa, West and Central African and North Africa, respectively (UNAIDS, 2013). Without treatment, PLWHA in need are highly vulnerable to complications. Unchecked viral replication increases the risk of further HIV transmission and the risk of death among PLWHA (UNAIDS, 2013). The gap among children is wider with the highest (94%) in North Africa. When treatment is denied, it is tantamount to denying the affected PLWHA the right to life, right to health and equal opportunity. Gaps in the treatment of PLWHA also pose a tremendous public health challenge to the entire population. There are also measures that will improve demand when the supply is steady. The right to privacy and confidentiality are very crucial to cut the number of HIV-related deaths; by respecting those rights, more people will feel safe to access counseling and testing services, and eventual enrolment for treatment for those that are positive. The PLWHA also deserve fair treatment and a non-judgmental attitude from health workers and the general public.

References

Amzat, J. (2015). The question of autonomy in maternal health: a rights-based consideration. *Journal of Bioethical Inquiry, 15*(2), 283–293. doi:10.1007/s11673-015-9607-y.

Azevedo, M. A. (2010). Right as entitlements, and rights as claims. *Veritas, 55*(1), 164–182.

De Neve, J., Fink, G., Subramanian, S. V., Moyo, S., Bor, J. (2015). Length of secondary schooling and risk of HIV infection in Botswana: evidence from a natural experiment. *Lancet Global Health, 3*, e470–e477.

Florin, D. (2004). Public involvement in health care. *BMJ, 328*, 159–161. doi:10.1136/bmj. 328.7432.159.

Flowers, N. (1999). *Human rights here and now: Celebrating the Universal Declaration of Human Rights*. Minneapolis: Human Rights Educators' Network, Amnesty International.

Gruskin, S., & Tarantola, D. (2002). Human rights and HIV/AIDS. http://hivinsite.ucsf.edu/InSite?page=kb-08-01-07. Accessed 12 May 2016.

Heise, L., Germain, A. and Pitanguy, J. (1994). Violence against women: the hidden health burden. World Bank Discussion Paper, No 255. Washington, DC: The World Bank.

Hunt, P. (2006). The human right to the highest attainable standard of health: new opportunities and challenges. *Transaction of the Royal Society of Tropical Medicine and Hygiene, 100*(7), 603–607.

Hunt, P., & Backman, G. (2008). Health systems and the right to the highest attainable standard of health. *Health and Human Rights: An Interna tional Journal, 10*(1), 81–92.

Karlsen, S., Say, L., Souza, J., Hogue, C. J., Calles, D. L., Gülmezoglu, A. M., Raine, R. (2011). The relationship between maternal education and mortality among women giving birth in health care institutions: analysis of the cross sectional WHO Global Survey on Maternal and Perinatal Health. *BMC Public Health, 11*, 606. doi:10.1186/1471-2458-11-606.

Kingston, L. N., Cohen, E. F., Morley, C. P. (2010). Limitations on universality: the "right to health" and the necessity of legal nationality. *BMC International Health and Human Right, 10*, 11. doi:10.1186/1472-698X-10-11.

Lamm, R. (1998). The case against making healthcare a "right". *American Bar Association: Defending Liberty Pursuing Justice, 25*(4), 8–11.

Leary, V. A. (1994). The right to health in international human rights law. *Health and Human Rights, 1*(1), 24–56.

Loefler, I. J. P. (1999). Health care is a human right" is a meaningless and devastating manifesto. *British Medical Journal, 318*(7200), 1766.

Maleche, A., & Day, E. (2011). *Traditional cultural practices and HIV: reconciling culture and human rights*. Working Paper for the Third Meeting of the Technical Advisory Group of the Global Commission on HIV and the Law, 7–9 July 2011.

Mann, J. M., Gostin, L., Gruskin, S., Brennan, T., Lazzarini, Z., Fineberg, H. V. (1994). Health and human rights. *Health and Human Rights, 1*(1), 6–23.

Mulumba, M., Kabanda, D., Nassuna, V. (2010). Constitutional provisions for the right to health in east and southern Africa; EQUINET Discussion Paper 81. Centre for Health, Human Rights and Development, Regional Network for Equity in Health in East and Southern Africa (EQUINET), Harare, Zimbabwe.

Pieterse, M. (2014). *Can rights cure? The impact of human rights litigation on South Africa's health system*. Pretoria: Pretoria Law Press.

Quane, H. (2012). A further dimension to the interdependence and indivisibility of human rights? Recent developments concerning the rights of indigenous peoples. *Harvard Human Rights Journal, 25*, 49–83.

Rendtorff, J. D. (2002). Basic ethical principles in European bioethics and biolaw: autonomy, dignity, integrity and vulnerability—towards a foundation of bioethics and biolaw. *Medicine, Health Care, and Philosophy, 5*(3), 235–244.

Sen, A. (2003). Missing women—revisited: reduction in female mortality has been counterbalanced by sex selective abortions. *BMJ, 327*, 1297–1298.

Singh, J. A., Govender, M., Mills, E. J. (2007). Do human rights matter to health? *Lancet, 370*, 521–27.

Staniszewska, S., Herron-Marx, S., Mockford, C. (2008). Measuring the impact of patient and public involvement: the need for an evidence base. *International Journal for Quality in Health Care, 20*(6), 373–374.

UNAIDS (2013). *Access to antiretroviral therapy in Africa: status report on progress towards the 2015 targets*. Geneva: UNAIDS.

UNAIDS (2014). *Reduction of HIV-related stigma and discrimination*. Geneva: Joint United Nations Programme on HIV/AIDS.

World Health Organization [WHO] (1948). *Constitution of the WHO*. Geneva: WHO.

WHO (1978). Declaration of Alma-Ata, International Conference on Primary Health Care, Alma-Ata, USSR, 6–12 September 1978.

WHO (2016). The Right to Health. http://www.ohchr.org/Documents/Publications/Factsheet31. pdf. Accessed 12 May 2016.

World Bank (2011). *World Development Report 2012: gender equality and development*. Washington, DC: World Bank.

Chapter 3
Healthcare Delivery Systems

3.1 Introduction

In general, the field of political economy of health has been concerned with how to relate socio-economic systems to healthcare performance. It is generally assumed that the healthcare system (either capitalist or socialist) has profound implications for the health indicators of any nation. The argument is also in line with the social production of health and illness. Basically, socialist or capitalist healthcare system provides a general comparative terrain for those interested in social production of health, as both of them are fraught with strengths and weaknesses. In reality, there is hardly a country with a pure socialist or a pure capitalist healthcare system; only one system is predominant over the other. For instance, USA is often cited as predominantly capitalist, but still has some safety nets provided by the government for certain segments of the population such as the poor and the elderly. There is also the emergence of neoliberal drive in healthcare, but it shares a number of similarities with the old capitalist system. This is why in this chapter, the discussion will be around capitalist-cum-neoliberal (c-cum-n) healthcare system.

The debate is ongoing as to the best form a healthcare system should take to guarantee the best care for the general population worldwide. Most African countries tend to practice what is called the two-tier healthcare system, a mix of both public and private provision of healthcare. The two-tier system is fraught with its own peculiarities and challenges. It is evident that the mixed system has helped but has not been able to eliminate the disease burden in Africa. While some societies are faring relatively better (in some aspects), majority of the countries face high disease burden, which further impend their socio-economic development.

The continent of Africa (in particular, sub-Saharan Africa) still battles with how best to tackle its excessively high disease burden. Because of systemic failures the continent has faced in tackling this challenge over the years, Africa is still not a healthy continent, despite the mixed system. With an extremely high

© Springer International Publishing AG 2018

J. Amzat, O. Razum, *Towards a Sociology of Health Discourse in Africa*,
DOI 10.1007/978-3-319-61672-8_3

proportion of the population living in poverty, there is still a large dependence on out-of-pocket contributions and user fees that place the greatest burden on the poorest members of society (KPMG-Africa, 2012). While there have been improvements in global health indicators, progress is slower in Africa. The critical question is which healthcare system works and why. The basic aim here is to introduce the three major patterns of healthcare systems (capitalist, socialist and mixed systems), focusing on their strengths and weaknesses.

3.2   Capitalist-Cum-Neoliberal Healthcare System

Capitalism emerged as a distinct socio-political and economic system following the industrial revolution of the eighteenth century. Since then it has been the mainstay of socio-economic system all over the world, although it has been severely criticized. Capitalism simply means a socio-political and economic system that allows for private ownership of property and means of production. Scott (2006, p. 1) defined capitalism "as an economic system where private actors are allowed to own and control the use of property in accord with their own interests, and where the invisible hand of the pricing mechanism coordinates supply and demand in markets in a way that is automatically in the best interests of society." In other words, capitalism "is an indirect system of governance based on a complex and continually evolving political bargain in which private actors are empowered by a political authority to own and control the use of property for private gain subject to a set of laws and regulations" (Scott, 2006, p. 4).

Neoliberalism represents a resurgence of the old capitalism or laissez-faire, although not usually used interchangeably. The term is not new, having been coined by Alexander Rüstow in 1938 to describe a new form of economic movement that is based on free enterprise (Hartwich, 2009). Most capitalist systems tends towards neo-liberal perspectives, which share some features with the capitalist system, including privatization, deregulation, free trade, structural adjustment programs (SAPs) and decentralization. Proponents of neoliberalism believe that the state should use its power to keep the market as free as possible from intervention, while creating a stable socio-economic and political environment for market operators to function. Like capitalism, it is an individualist system, which plays down the role of solidarity in healthcare. Structural Adjustment Programs imply that the government should reduce its spending and allow market forces to determine price and buffer its own shortcomings (where they arise) in order to provide best quality services (in this case, healthcare) to the general population. Many African nations have subscribed to the International Monetary Fund (IMF)-recommended SAPs, creating a kind of neo-liberalism, and consequently, austerity.

The capitalist-cum-neoliberal (c-cum-n) healthcare system is a form that is deregulated, that is free of strict government control and thus allows for private individuals to operate in the provision of the healthcare system. It has also been called different names including market-based or libertarian healthcare systems.

This system is a typical "fee for service" system, where the patient directly pays the doctor who provides the service. In advanced cases, payment is made through premiums to health insurance companies, which later reimburse the physicians. The primary foundation is that the patient gets what he/she pays for. The three major components are that:

1. The healthcare system is operated for a private profit; since individuals invest in it as a business, it is important that it is not operated at a loss so as to remain in business.
2. Private actors make decisions regarding location, supply, demand, price and distribution of healthcare facility/services determined by the market forces in the free market. Private actors decide where the healthcare facility will be located in a way that will attract demand as much as possible and ensure profit maximization.
3. The private healthcare providers are governed by sets rules that regulate their activities in the pursuance of their interests.

3.2.1 Strengths of the C-cum-N Healthcare System

The c-cum-n healthcare system has survived over the years because of its strengths in meeting the healthcare needs of the population. Many scholars have argued that capitalism, due to its attributes, is responsible for the tremendous success recorded over the years in healthcare, especially in the development of new technologies (see Ackerly, Valvered, Diener, Dossary, & Schulman, 2008; Lehoux, Miller, Daudelin, & Urbach, 2016). Many countries of the world operate a partially market-based health system along with socialized medicine. Some countries are predominantly capitalist in nature. The c-cum-n system is congruent with democratic ethics (including freedom of choice and equity). This is because it is devoid of stringent measures in term of access to healthcare because it is based on a free market system.

3.2.1.1 Freedom of Choice

In c-cum-n healthcare system, there is freedom of choice. It is generally argued that there is no "alternative" to freedom. In open market-based systems, there is usually an influx of care-providers. This opens the market for the consumers to choose from various providers in order to access desired care. The choice available is not limited. The argument is that a universal entitlement to healthcare can be grounded in the liberty principle (Sachs, 2008). This is the greatest strength of the c-cum-n healthcare system, and it is in strong contrast to the provisions in a controlled system; where citizens are limited to accessing healthcare through the public-funded institutions, allowing them to only have access to what is provided by the single provider: the government.

3.2.1.2 Innovation and Creativity

The c-cum-n system encourages innovation and creativity. Therefore, provision of healthcare is competitive in the open market to enhance dynamism and ingenuity that will lead to better services. This is why in c-cum-n systems, medical care of high sophistication is usually available. This is highly beneficial to the consumers, as the quality of care will continue to grow; and it will be self-sustaining. This will ensure adequate value for money spent on healthcare. For the investors to make profits, they have to provide quality services in a competitive market, or those who provide superior care will attract more consumers than their counterparts.

3.2.1.3 Sense of Responsibility

Another major argument in favor of the c-cum-n system is the belief that it promotes a sense of responsibility on the part of the consumers. The world is now witnessing an increase in lifestyle diseases. It is assumed that when individual are aware of their responsibility regarding the consequences of their actions, they will reduce their unhealthy behavior. Costs of treatment of tobacco- and alcohol-related diseases can discourage people from smoking and excessive drinking. While holding individuals accountable for their choices in the context of healthcare is controversial (Cappelen & Norheim, 2005), it can actually shape health-related behavior and choices, which might not be obtainable in other systems. Perhaps, diseases that are related to sexual behavior (e.g., HIV), dietary behavior (e.g., obesity) and other lifestyle-related health disease conditions might be reduced.

3.2.1.4 Efficiency

The c-cum-n healthcare system of care promotes efficiency. It is usually a coordinated system of stakeholders pursuing self-interest within the limits of the law. Therefore, they try to channel all resources (technology, capital and labor) in a manner that would yield better proceeds. The market forces (regarding healthcare) ensure that resources are distributed according to consumer preferences. The providers avoid waste as much as possible to improve competitiveness and adequate provision of services. At the same time, health providers respond to changes in consumer preferences and adhere to best practices. This is a prerequisite for quality of care, which in a market-based system is fundamental to the sustainability of the system. Beyond the price, quality is also important to consumers. To ensure efficiency and high quality, health institutions will aim to acquire the latest technologies and uphold best practices in order to have the best share of the market.

3.2.1.5 Equality Based on Ability-to-Pay

There is also a form of equality in accessing healthcare that c-cum-n promotes. This form is predicated on the notion that every citizen is on the same playing ground. Levies are attached to services not to persons. Individuals exercise freedom of choice based on available resources. So far as individuals have the means, the standard of care is relatively similar. The individual also reserves the right to complain or even sue in case of perceived discrimination or poor quality of services. Protection of rights is a democratic value, which is also not contrary to the c-cum-n healthcare system.

3.2.2 Weaknesses of the C-cum-N Healthcare System

The capitalist healthcare system has been widely criticized, primarily with the argument that healthcare is an essential need, which should not be based on a market system.

3.2.2.1 Commodification of Health

In a capitalist system, everything is a commodity, which everyone should be able to pay for and enjoy. A c-cum-n healthcare system is also commoditized (turned in to a commodity), hence it can be bought by those who have the means to do so. Those that have been pauperized by the same system might not be able to access healthcare. In most African countries, for instance, more than half of the population lives below the poverty-line, making access to healthcare in a market system unattainable. Even though there is equality based on ability to pay, not everyone has such ability.

3.2.2.2 Inequalities in Disease Burden

The c-cum-n healthcare system often leads to growing inequalities in disease burden. As a consequence of commodification, and because of high poverty levels, the disadvantaged population will continue to bear the greater brunt of the illness burden. Poverty increases vulnerability to diseases through a complex web of (unfavorable) determinants of health, such shortage of food and poor housing and working conditions. In general, c-cum-n healthcare systems are less likely than other types of healthcare systems to produce equality in health outcomes among all strata of a society.

3.2.2.3   Inequalities in Care

In addition to inequalities in disease burden, c-cum-n can lead to inequalities in care. Rylko-Bauer and Farmer (2002, p. 476) observed that "allowing market forces to dictate the shape of healthcare delivery ensures that inequalities in care will continue to grow and modern medicine will become increasingly adept at managing inequality rather than managing (providing) care." It is stressed that for-profit healthcare institutions fail to fulfill their obligations to do their fair share in providing healthcare to the poor and so exacerbate the problem of access to healthcare (Buchanan, 1987). In the African context, where access to care has always been a major challenge, deregulation (as exists in a c-cum-n system) would further reinforce the inequalities in access to care. Health inequalities magnify the effects of general social inequalities in the society. The c-cum-n healthcare system makes healthcare less affordable to vulnerable populations (especially the lower class). It makes quality care a luxury for the less privileged, hence, increasing morbidity and mortality in those groups.

3.2.2.4   Increasing Cost of Care

The challenge of diminishing returns and escalating costs is crucial in a capitalist setting. It has been argued, even in advanced capitalist systems, that the skyrocketing cost of healthcare is no longer commensurate with the actual healthcare (see Waitzkin, 1981). Waitzkin (1981) generally faulted the capitalist claim that the general improvement in health conditions in industrialized countries is a result of capitalist advancement in healthcare. What is evident is that, particularly in a c-cum-n system, an increase in healthcare costs is felt keenly by the general population, who have no alternative but to pay higher prices for this essential and indispensable good. At least, there must be profit maximization in order to keep the investors in the market.

3.2.2.5   Minimal Social Benefits

In a c-cum-n system, in order to ensure competiveness, the principle of non-interference from the government is a necessary norm. The market forces must be at play in order to create a conducive environment for investors. The main role of the government is not invested in the direct provision of healthcare, but rather to create a supportive environment for everyone to participate in the market. This hands-off governmental approach could lead to a reduction in social safety nets (in the form of social welfare) overall. For instance, in the USA, government healthcare assistance is limited to the vulnerable populations of the elderly and the poor. Efforts to expand the scope of the subsidized care have always met with strong opposition from strongest proponents of capitalism.

3.2.2.6 Poor Patient-Practitioner Relations

A market-based health system with profit maximization can jeopardize the quality of the patient-physician relationship (Buchanan, 1987). It is usually a form of calculative relationship where both parties try as much as possible to maximize benefits. In general, due to professional power, charges must be paid irrespective of how the patients feel about it. The trust between the parties is likely diminished because the patients often feel the physician is motivated more by profit, not for altruistic motives. Buchanan (1987) attested that "profit seeking in medicine will damage the physician-patient relationship, creating conflicts of interest that will diminish the quality of care and erode patients' trust in their physicians and the public's trust in the medical profession." The ethical implications of the commodification of healthcare are complex because healthcare becomes a "product" supplied by the healthcare "provider," resulting in the possibility of tension between professional ethics and marketplace strategies (Rowe & Moodley, 2013). This is a real possibility, as physicians might then be viewed as businessmen rather than as care-givers.

3.2.2.7 Growing Medicalization

Unnecessary medicalization is a growing problem in medicine. Conrad (2005, p. 3) observed that medicalization involves defining any type of problem in medical terms, usually as an illness or disorder, or using a medical intervention to treat it (Conrad, 2005, p. 3). It has been observed that there is close link between "medicalization and the commodification of social maladies as disease and illness" (Kennedy, 2015, p. 211). Medicalization involves the medical gaze shifting from patients to the general population, or from illness to life itself (Illich, 1975). To create a greater market, and ultimately more profits, more "health" commodities need to be created. The world is witnessing the medicalization of sexuality (the rise of sexual enhancement drugs even for healthy individuals) and medicalization of beauty (rising cosmetic procedures). In a capitalist system, this will continue to expand unabated, in order to generate more market products.

3.3 The Socialist-Cum-Socialized (S-cum-S) Healthcare System

Socialism is a socio-economic and political system in which the means of production, distribution, and exchange are owned and regulated by the government. By this measure, socialism is the opposite of capitalism. Socialism is a kind of common ownership of (state) property, since all resources are administered on behalf of the people by the government. Socialist healthcare systems are also in line with public ownership, regulation and distribution of the health services in a way that will ensure universal access. Although socialized medicine or healthcare is based on the same principles of socialism, it is not exclusive to socialist socio-political and economic systems (the prime examples of this are the UK and Canada). In Africa, Tanzania experimented with a socialist system from 1961 to the early 1980s (Bjerk, 2010), including a socialist healthcare system. As envisaged by Loewy (1997), it was a single-tiered socialist healthcare system supported by general tax revenue and administered by a central body. However, the system ultimately collapsed. Like market-based healthcare systems, the socialist system has strengths and weaknesses.

3.3.1 Strengths of the Socialist Healthcare System

The socialist healthcare system has attracted a good deal of attention, due, among other things, to its promise of universal access and equity.

3.3.1.1 Universal Coverage

In a socialist system, healthcare is an entitlement of all members of the community, instead of being something available without cost only to those below a certain income range. Universal coverage means that everyone who needs services should get those services in appropriate quality. Therefore, free access to needed healthcare is a legitimate expectation for all members of the community (Loewy, 1997). There is no demographic criterion defining access to care. Every citizen, irrespective of age, sex and other socio-demographic attributes, has the right to healthcare. This main feature makes socialized medicine acceptable to many advocates of "health for all." Healthcare is viewed as a social good, which is collectively financed and available to all.

3.3.1.2 Equality in Access to Care

Another major strength is egalitarian nature in accessing care. There is equality in access to care. The ease at which people access healthcare is relatively even. Since, there is common/public ownership of the healthcare system, there is equality (i.e., no discrimination). Unlike in the market-based system where equality is guaranteed only if the patient has the ability-to-pay, in the socialist system, every citizen has the right to healthcare because it is publicly financed. Willingness to access the service is a major criterion in utilizing healthcare services under the socialist system. This is a point that makes socialized medicine attractive to many people.

3.3.1.3 Affordability

The main point here is that out-of-pocket payment for healthcare is eliminated as healthcare is financed through public revenue. Hence, healthcare is affordable to all patients. One of the major problems in accessing healthcare is cost of care (especially direct cost). It is a major problem affecting access to care in Africa. But with the socialized healthcare, such problem is minimized or eliminated through state intervention (i.e., by direct bearing healthcare costs). A socialized medicine will help those living below the poverty-line to access care. In most health discourse including access to healthcare and UHC, the question of affordability is predominant. The financial barrier has been a fundamental issue in access to care in Africa especially because of high level of poverty. There must also be financial protection. This is why there is gradual campaign against out-of-pocket payment, which is rampant in Africa.

3.3.2 Weaknesses of the Socialist Healthcare System

Despite these strengths, socialist medicine has also been the subject of criticism. Some of these grounds will be briefly discussed.

3.3.2.1 Monopolistic in Nature

Socialism is often equated with the use of force; so is socialized medicine. Use of force or lack of freedom of choice is inimical to the doctrine of democracy. There is no freedom of choice as everyone has to patronize the healthcare provided by the government, and complies with all the measures instituted by the same government. The quality of care, distribution of health services, location of facilities and modalities for accessing care (which might include compulsory registration with public insurance and payment of taxes) are determined or enforced by a single player, leaving citizens with no other alternatives. This is monopolistic in nature, and might not yield the desired outcomes in terms of essential needs such as healthcare. As previously mentioned, one advantage of multiple-player healthcare is that consumer will select from different plans and providers, and will have opportunity to switch from one to the other in case of any dissatisfaction. With the socialist system, opportunity for selection and switching might not be available.

3.3.2.2 Rationing and Shortages

Socialist healthcare promotes rationing and shortages. It is often not feasible to provide comprehensive coverage. Most often, only the most essential services are defined and provided. This reflects a utilitarian perspective of maximization of benefit to the maximum number of people instead of aspiring for total coverage.

What the state defines as "essential healthcare" may not be acceptable to all. Invariably, minority groups with special needs will not find the care they need, or will have to pay out-of-pocket or travel outside the country to seek treatment. For example, in SSA there could be over concentration on malaria and other preventable diseases, which provide maximum benefit to the majority, rather than some chronic diseases, which would gulp large some of money but only for the benefit of the minority. This could be term as discrimination in healthcare provision; universal coverage is achieved, but at the cost of comprehensive care.

3.3.2.3 Inefficiency in Service Delivery

Apart from lack of comprehensive care, there could also be inefficiency in service delivery. A single player often dictates the pace of every aspect of healthcare. When there is no market competition, public expenditure may escalate. In a situation in which inadequate budgeting for healthcare prevails, there be could chaos in the system as demand increases in the face of limited supply of services. Market competition should ordinarily drive prices down without the need for price fixing. Limited resources available might not be judiciously utilized to get the best outcome with minimal expenditure. Therefore, apart from shortages, wastages may also arise.

3.3.2.4 Delay in Care

Long waiting period in accessing care is also a major downside of the socialist healthcare system. This is because everyone turns to a single provider; the limit of the healthcare system might be over-stretched. The health workers might overwork without commensurate incentive/motivation. This will create a long waiting period for some procedures/services, and long waiting hours for every contact with the health facility. In this case, providers may sacrifice the quality of services or may provide only a limited number of services. In Africa, where there is already shortage of health workers and health facilities, overcrowding in the few health facilities is expected, which will definitely and adversely impact access to and quality of care. Even with the availability of private providers, the situation in public hospitals is that of long waiting period and limited services.

The foregoing discussion about the c-cum-n and s-cum-s shows the inherent strengths and weaknesses of the two systems. Neither system is perfect, or could be a perfect solution to the healthcare challenges of every nation. In addition, the effectiveness of the system might also depend on the certain national factors and the kind of regulations put in place. The fact remains that whether socialist/ socialized or c-cum-n healthcare system, no nation practicing either of the two is free from healthcare challenges. The essence of this discussion is not to make specific judgment about which nation is faring better than the other. In order to resolve healthcare issues, some nations opt for a combined strategy: a mix of socialist and capitalist system known as the two-tier healthcare system.

3.4 Two-Tier Healthcare System

The two-tier system allows for both private and public players in the provision of healthcare services. In other words, it is a system which allows for a public healthcare system that provides care for all citizens coupled with a parallel system whereby individuals can purchase additional or specialized care (Smith, 2007). Thus, it is a mix of both capitalist and socialist healthcare systems. It has been argued that this mix would provide a way of counterbalancing the weaknesses of one system with the strengths of the other. This should then provide what is close to a perfect system of healthcare delivery. In Africa, the two-tier system stems from the non-aligned movement, thus allowing for a dual system to operate in order to create more opportunities in terms of preference and quality of care. In most instances in Africa, public institutions provide not completely free, but rather subsidized healthcare.

3.4.1 Strengths of the Two-Tier Healthcare System

In contrast to a one-tier system, there is an open alternative from which the consumer can choose. As the public and private tiers run side by side, those individuals who are not satisfied with one tier can switch to another in a drive to get better care.

3.4.1.1 Comprehensive Services from Both Tiers

Two-tier system ensures comprehensive services, which can be obtained in either of the systems. This is simply possible because services that cannot be obtained in the public tier might be accessed in the private tier. This ensures that all levels of care are catered for within the same system. This notion of comprehensive services might be different from comprehensive coverage in a single tier system. At least those who require higher level of care, who are able to pay, can obtain it in the alternative tier. In this case, it takes one system to complement the services provided by the other.

3.4.1.2 Combined Strategy

As previously observed, two-tier system offsets the shortcoming of one system with the strength of the other. The strengths and weaknesses of both capitalist and socialist have been previously explained. One of the dreams of the two-tier system is to upset the inherent weaknesses in any of the systems. This is a combined-strategy that has been the core of healthcare system in most developing countries especially in Africa. The extent to which this has really worked is still a matter of debate, but it still remains clear that it a parallel system of care with some competition, complementarity and conflict.

3.4.1.3   Availability of Social Benefits

The system caters for the needs of the less privileged as a well as that of the upper class. While the general public can easily opt for the affordable public healthcare services, other can access private care which might be more expensive, faster and of higher quality. This allows for a shorter waiting period, for those who can afford it. This is evident in most African countries, as those in the upper wealth quintile might even travel abroad to access better care. Most of the governments have been trying to invest on primary healthcare system, which should provide basic/essential care to teeming poor and the general public at large. Sometimes, free medical care is provided to improve the health indicators of the country. For instance, maternal and childcare, treatment of HIV and TB, and family planning services have been largely subsidized in several African countries.

3.4.1.4   Better Management of Public Expenditure

The two-tier system should lead to better management of public expenditure. In order to cut the high costs of healthcare, only a two-tier system with explicitly limited public guarantees and optional privately financed health services seems acceptable (Breyer & Kliemt, 2015). The private tier should be able to complement the efforts of the government in providing care, and bear a substantial part of the financial burden which otherwise would have accrued to the government alone. In some cases, government only concentrates in providing essential care (usually primary care) while the private tier provides secondary care. The situation is not that demarcated in most African countries, as there is no sharp line in terms of type of care.

3.4.2   Weaknesses of the Two-tier Healthcare System

It is generally observed that the two healthcare sectors (public and private) are distinct in terms of form, modality of disbursing services and ideology of care (Ghoshal, 2015). Therefore, mixing them often complicates issues. As it will later be observed, there could be linkages often difficult to resolve. This is also a case of clash of ideology and differential challenges created by bi-directional approach in healthcare.

3.4.2.1 Special Privilege to the Privileged

In the two-tier system, inequality is further perpetuated. Wealth will definitely allow some patients to access medical services faster with higher quality, while other with similar needs might not enjoy the timely and quality care (see Krohmal and Emanuel, 2009). In poor countries, some might die on the waiting list for a simple procedure. This is evident in the education sector in several African countries, where children of the upper class are now abandoning the public schools, for only the children of the poor to attend. Over time, the inequality in morbidity and mortality will be obvious. There is tendency for the private health sector to be better organized and more efficient, due to their drive to recruit more patients and make profits.

3.4.2.2 Undue Linkages

In most African countries, linkages between the systems are evident. It is often the norm for physicians to shift their time and other public resources to the private sector. Referrals are often made to the private sector for those who desire timely care and who can pay for it. The same physicians operating in the public institutions often have private hospitals where they deliver better and faster services. This often threatens the service delivery in the public sector. This is apart from cases of diversion of public resources to the private sector. For instance, insecticide treated-bednet meant to be freely distributed at public institutions found their way to the private medicine stores (Amzat, 2011). In many cases, publicly funded health services are limited, inefficient, and, in many situations, deliberately undermined for the gains of the private sector.

3.4.2.3 Overstretched Public Institutions

In developing countries, the preference for the public-funded is higher because it is often cheaper. This accounts for the persistence of waiting hours and period. Especially in countries where the majority live below the poverty-line, there is relatively high patronage of the public health institutions, which unfortunately, are limited in number of facilities, staff and capacities. The poor ill are marked by their low economic buying power, which often pushes them to access only the public healthcare sector, in which costs of treatment are subsidized by the state (Ghoshal, 2015).

3.4.2.4 Double Cost

Cost of care might also increase as people might double register for both public and private sector. Since there is duplication of healthcare provision, in the quest for better services, many individuals will register at both tiers resulting in high costs. Not only at the individual level, the cost of care might also increase at the level of the government. Demand for public health services will definitely increase due to preference for the public institution and as a right for the taxpayers.

3.4.2.5 Unequal Access

There could be discrimination, as those in formal and government employment may be better-covered compare to those in the informal sector. This is evident in Nigeria, as the NHIS mainly covers those in the formal sector, and the country must struggle with how to cover the teeming poor and rural dwellers. Some individuals benefit from the public tax, while others who should also have the right to the benefits are systematically denied. This is no justice in healthcare provision if it is not universal and on equal terms. It is also possible that some segments of the population might be under-served.

3.4.2.6 Urban Bias

The rural areas might still be largely underserved with healthcare services. It is expected that there will be a higher concentration of private healthcare ventures in urban and peri-urban areas, where the majority of the middle and upper classes reside (see Ghoshal, 2015). The venture is meant to make profit and will likely concentrate where consumers who are willing and able to pay reside. The urban bias will further be perpetuated in distribution of healthcare services. This has been the major challenge over the years in most African countries. Ghoshal (2015) observed that "the growing glamour of the private healthcare sector has led to the formation of a distinct class of patients—the affluent ill, with those outside this ambit constituting the class of the non-affluent or the poor ill" who normally wait at the public health institution.

References

Ackerly, D. C., Valvered, A. M., Diener, L. W., Dossary, K. L., Schulman, K. A. (2008). Fueling innovation in medical devices (and beyond): venture capital in health care. *Health Affairs, 28*(1), w68–w75.

Amzat, J. (2011). Assessing the progress of malaria control in Nigeria. *World Health and Population, 12*(3), 42–51.

Bjerk, P. K. (2010). Sovereignty and socialism in Tanzania: the historiography of an African State. *History in Africa, 37*, 275–319.

Breyer, F., & Kliemt, H. (2015). "Priority of Liberty" and the design of a two-tier health care system. *Journal of Medicine and Philosophy, 40*(2), 137–151. doi:10.1093/jmp/jhu076.

Buchanan, A. E. (1987). The profit motive in medicine. *Journal of Medicine and Philosophy*, *12*(1), 1–35.

Cappelen, A. W., & Norheim, O. F. (2005). Responsibility in health care: a liberal egalitarian approach. *Journal of Medical Ethics*, *31*, 476–480.

Conrad, P. (2005). The shifting engines of medicalization. *Journal of Health and Social Behavior*, *46*, 3–14.

Ghoshal, R. (2015). What ails India's two-tiered healthcare system? A philosophical enquiry. *Indian Journal of Medical Ethics*, *12*(1), 25–29.

Hartwich, O. M. (2009). Neoliberalism: the genesis of a political swearword. CIS Occasional Paper 114, Centre for Independent Studies. Sydney, New South Wales.

Illich, I. (1975). The medicalization of life. *Journal of Medical Ethics*, *1*, 73–77.

Kennedy, P. (2015). The contradictions of capitalist healthcare system. *Critique: Journal of Socialist Theory*, *43*(2), 211–231.

KPMG-Africa (2012). The state of healthcare in Africa. Johannesburg, South Africa.

Krohmal, B. J., & Emanuel, E. J. (2009). Tiers without tears: the ethics of a two-tier health care system. In B. Steinbock (Ed.). *The Oxford handbook of bioethics*. Oxford: Oxford University Press.

Lehoux, P., Miller, F. A., Daudelin, G., Urbach, D. R. (2016). How venture capitalists decide which new medical technologies come to exist. *Science and Public Policy*, *43*(3), 375–385. doi:10.1093/scipol/scv051.

Loewy, E. H. (1997). What would a socialist health care system look like? A sketch. *Health Care Analysis*, *5*, 3195–204.

Rowe, K., & Moodley, K. (2013). Patients as consumers of health care in South Africa: the ethical and legal implications. *BMC Medical Ethics*, *14*, 15. doi:10.1186/1472-6939-14-15.

Rylko-Bauer, B., & Farmer, P. (2002). Managed care or managed inequality? A call for critiques of market-based medicine. *Medical Anthropology Quarterly*, *16*(4), 476–502.

Sachs, B. (2008). The liberty principle and universal healthcare. *Kennedy Institute of Ethics Journal*, *18*(2), 149–172.

Scott, B. R. (2006). The political economy of capitalism. Harvard Business School, Harvard Working Paper, www.hbs.edu/faculty/Publication%20Files/07-037.pdf. Accessed 4 May 2016.

Smith, E. R. (2007). A two-tier healthcare system: is there anything new? *Canadian Journal of Cardiology*, *23*(11), 915–916.

Waitzkin, H. (1981). A marxist analysis of the healthcare systems of advanced capitalist societies. In L. Eisenberg, A. Kleinman (Eds.). *The relevance of social science for medicine* (pp. 333–369). Dordrecht: Springer.

Chapter 4
Health Financing and Insurance in Africa

4.1 Introduction

Healthcare, like any service, requires funding to succeed. Healthcare is funded by different nations in various ways, but it usually involves some combination of governmental support, insurance company support, and individual out-of-pocket payments. The individual and the society play collaborative pivotal roles in health management. Most societies finance the healthcare system focusing on population health, i.e., to ensure overall wellbeing of the citizens.

The chapter starts with some notes on the state of health financing in Africa and later explains health insurance, which involves pooling risks with others in order to spread the cost of healthcare. Types of health insurance are discussed—social insurance, private for profit, private-non-profit and community-based health insurance (CBHI). An ideal health insurance helps to curb cost escalation and to improve quality and coverage of healthcare. However, health insurance does not yet cover large proportion of the population in many Africa countries. The national health insurance schemes in developing countries still face a number of challenges despite the benefits they promote. The fundamental argument has always been that there is a need to increase the coverage of health insurance and government needs to increase their health expenditure in order to achieve the goal of equitable access to healthcare for all.

4.2 The State of Healthcare Financing in Africa

The main source of healthcare finance in African countries is the national budget, supported by other sources such as the private sector and foreign aid. There is always clamor for the state to increase the healthcare budget in order to achieve targeted health goals. This is because the problems of low levels of public funding and high

© Springer International Publishing AG 2018   51
J. Amzat, O. Razum, *Towards a Sociology of Health Discourse in Africa*,
DOI 10.1007/978-3-319-61672-8_4

out-of-pocket payment are still prevalent in Africa: as at 2012, Sub-Saharan Africa spent 6.1% of its total gross domestic products (GDP) on health, far less than the 9.5% of GDP that the countries of the Organization for Economic Co-operation and Development (OECD) spend on health (National Academy of Science, 2012). In 2009, low-income countries reportedly spent $25 per person on health versus the more than $4,600 per person spent in high-income countries. Per capita health spending was $83, less than 2% of the average spending in high-income countries (National Academy of Science, 2012). Data from other African countries show a wide variation in per capita spending on health. In 2014, spending ranged from US$7 in the Democratic Republic of Congo to US$511 in Equatorial Guinea (WHO, 2013). Apart from the amount of spending, another crucial point is how the funding is effectively or judiciously utilized to achieve health goals. The highest government expenditure on health in SSA is not near the average obtainable in the advanced countries. As previously mentioned, public spending is the major source of funding for health in Africa. While private and foreign aid also contribute, they are usually complementary and often far below the government spending. While some countries are gradually improving, although not yet commensurate to the target or expectation, many countries such as Angola, Benin, Cameroon, CAR, Ghana, Guinea Bissau, Kenya, Madagascar, Mali, Niger, and Zimbabwe are fairing very poorly despite facing enormous health challenges.

In terms of a spending benchmark, the Abuja Declaration by African countries promises to allocate at least 15% of the government budget to health in order to meet the healthcare challenges facing the region. There is also the recommendation of the High-Level Taskforce on Innovative International Financing for Health Systems (HLFT) to allocate at least US$44 per capital to deliver essential packages of health services. As of 2010, WHO reported that only Botswana, Rwanda and Zambia have been able to meet the Abuja target (WHO, 2013) (see Table 4.1). Furthermore, while Equatorial Guinea has the highest per capita health expenditure, the country has not met the Abuja target.

Table 4.1 Total health expenditure against GGHE/GGE

	GGHE/GGE more than 15%	GGHE/GGE less than 15%
Total health expenditure per capital more than US$44	Botswana, Rwanda, Zambia **(3 countries)**	Algeria, Angola, Cameroon, Cape Verde, Congo, Cote d'Ivoire, Equatorial Guinea, Gabon, Ghana, Guinea-Bissau, Lesotho, Mauritius, Namibia, Nigeria, Sao Tome and Principe, Senegal, Seychelles, South Africa, Swaziland, Uganda **(20 countries)**
Total health expenditure per capita less than US$44	Madagascar, Togo **(2 countries)**	Benin, Burkina Faso, Burundi, Central African Republic, Chad, Comoros, DRC, Eritrea, Ethiopia, Gambia, Guinea, Kenya, Liberia, Malawi, Mali, Mauritania, Mozambique, Niger, Sierra Leone, Tanzania **(20 countries)**

Source WHO (2013).
GGE, General Government Expenditure; GGHE, Government General Health Expenditure.

The prevailing budget insufficiency put the issues of universal healthcare coverage and access to health care in a state of uncertainty. Financial protection and the ability to afford health services are often elusive in many African countries, making it difficult to ensure financial protection or provide comprehensive services for the benefit of the citizens. At least in terms of finance, it is thus evident why the disease burden is high and access to healthcare is relatively poor in Africa. In several African countries, the health budget is far from meeting needs and targets. One major best practice in ensuring financial protection is through health insurance. This is why the next few subsection will examine issues relating to health insurance in Africa.

4.3   What is Health Insurance?

The word "insurance" comes from the word "insure" which means the act of entering into agreement which involves promises to pay somebody an amount of money or compensation in case of any form of tragedy including serious illness, accident, injury or death, damage or loss of property, based on agreed payment called premiums. The underlying principle is one of pooling (small) risks in (large) populations and paying out compensation from the collected premiums in case the insured event occurs. Health insurance involves pooling risks with others in order to spread costs of healthcare over time and thus protect against catastrophically expensive illness (Witter, 2000). Insurance can also be defined as "a device for reducing risk by combining a sufficient number of exposure units to make their loss collectively predictable. The predictable loss is then shared proportionally by all units in the combination." (Mehr, Cammack, & Rose, 1985). Insurance has also been defined as a means whereby groups (people facing similar risks) can come together for protection against certain financial (or social) losses (Dickson & John, 1987). Each individual transfers his/her risk to the club (in return for a fee). The "unlucky" few who suffer losses claim compensation from the fund. Similarly, Conn and Walford (1998) defined health insurance as a way of paying for some or all the cost of healthcare. It protects the insured persons from paying high treatment cost in the events of sickness. The overall essence of health insurance is to cover health risks, i.e., the probability or chances of occurrence or the management of occurrence of ill health—i.e., diseases, defect, infirmity or injury. The basic insurance process is as follows: a consumer makes a regular payment to a managing institution and healthcare providers. The outcome of the process is that the costs of individual consumers' healthcare needs are met (see Fig. 4.1).

From the different definitions, some facts about insurance are evident: Insurance is a risk transfer mechanism; it involves accumulation of funds (through premiums); it involves solidarity of people who similar bear loss or burden in event of loss or any form of damage; it is about indemnifying or compensating the insured that suffer losses; and it offers financial protection against uncertainties or tragedies.

Insurance is typically divided into two types: life insurance (which includes individual and group insurance) and general insurance (which includes a wide range of categories such as fire, accident, motor vehicle, oil and gas, work-men's

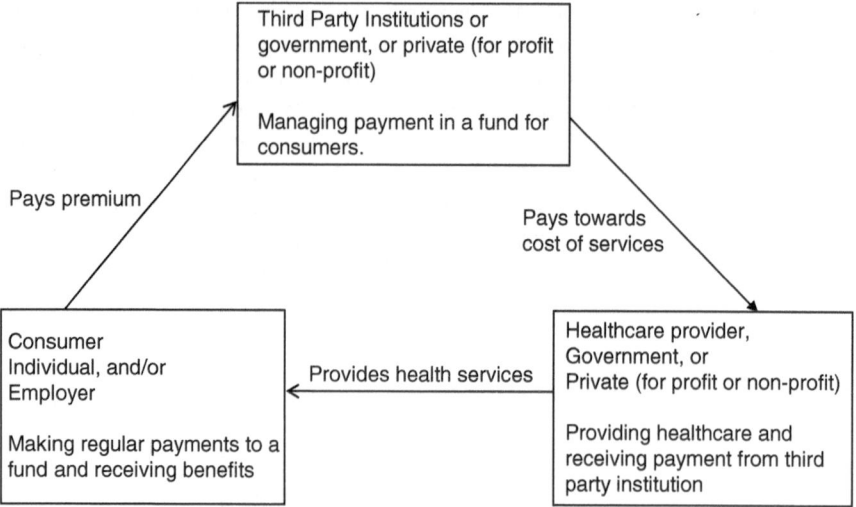

Fig. 4.1 The Health Insurance Process. *Source* Conn and Walford (1998)

compensation, goods-in-transit, marine, aviation, health insurance and miscellaneous insurance). Insurance involves risk pooling, a process by which people contribute to a general fund, from which they can be reimbursed if the need arises. This is the basis for all insurance funds. The costs of tragedy are then shared among members of the pool (thus risks are pooled) (Witter, 2000). In terms of health, the premiums are linked to the likelihood of an individual to incur health expenditures in the future (i.e., their expected ill-health, based on information about their past record, genetic factors or lifestyle), while in some cases, the solidarity principle is the main reason for health insurance irrespective of the likelihood of incurring health expenditure. This is called risk rating. Indemnity refers to the compensation made by the insurer to the assured in the occurrence of loss, damage or ill-health.

There are variations in the range of care provided under insurance. It may be limited to treatment for serious illness only or it may include routine treatments and preventive care, leading to different outcomes. Insurance policies often contain exemptions, that is, certain medications (preventive or treatment) are not covered. In some instances, additional premiums might be required if there are pre-existing medical conditions (especially chronic conditions). A pre-existing condition is a medical issue existing before an individual takes up a health insurance policy. The argument for charging higher premiums for pre-existing conditions is that insurance is meant to cover future unexpected occurrences, not events that have already occurred. One problem with this practice is that a (past) condition not adequately treated can lead to future complications. Hence, insurers who discriminate on the basis of pre-existing conditions have been criticized as inimical to standard ethics of financial protection in the face of illness.

4.3.1 Types of Health Insurance

There are three major types of health insurance that differ according to how they are funded: government (or public) health insurance (including Bismarck and Beveridge [premium- and tax-based respectively]), private insurance and community-based health insurance (CBHI).

4.3.1.1 Government Health Insurance Schemes

There are many kinds of government insurance schemes, often called social insurance. Social insurance, for example the National Health Insurance Scheme (NHIS), is available in many countries around the world. Social Insurance was first introduced in Europe at the end of the nineteenth century, spreading to Latin America in the 1930s, and to Eastern Europe and the former Soviet Union in the early 1990s. It has also been introduced in a number of developing countries, but often only covering civil servants or those in formal employment (Witter, 2000). It is usually compulsory for certain groups in the population and premiums are set according to income (ability to pay) rather than according to health risk (Conn & Walford, 1998). This is often referred to as the Bismarck, premium-based insurance model. The Bismarck model originates from Germany, where it is for the general public and not just for government workers. Since it is based on premium deducted directly from income/salary, it signifies a visible and clearly defined flow of funds into the health sector. Funds can be managed independent of the government (for example, by a constituted board) and protect the fund for health. The Bismarck model (as implemented in Germany) is a typical illustration of how private practice can effectively participate in a regulated health environment, since the German system is not solely for government workers. In most African countries, government insurance schemes mostly cover those in the public sector, or, in some cases, only government workers. Since it is based on premium deducted directly from income/salary.

In a government-controlled health insurance scheme, there could be a number of considerations in order to ensure adequate coverage. For instance, premium may be based on income threshold. This may mean that those earning below a certain threshold might pay less premium/tax to cover healthcare. The tax-based system is often referred to as the Beveridge model and is a progressive system based on income. The more an individual earns, the higher the tax. Healthcare is then funded from public revenue. The idea is to cover the less privileged or supplement premiums in care of the needy. The general aim of the government is to provide healthcare as welfare service. In most instances, this mostly covers essential or basic services for all enrollees. It is possible to combine the public insurance with a private one in order to have access to more services not covered or provided in the latter type.

The rationale of public health insurance is also clear in many nations. South Africa instituted NHI policy guided by social justice principles such as right to health and equity to ensure universal coverage (Naidoo, 2012). The Green paper was released in 2011 with a detailed plan to reform the healthcare system in South Africa by 2025 (Govender et al., 2013). Tunisia has one of the highest health insurance coverage rates in Africa with up to 90% of the population covered (Chahed & Arfa, 2014). The government ensures financial protection through the implementation of a two-tiered social protection system with health insurance and subsidized or free healthcare. The insurance scheme is funded through employee contributions and government-subsidized coverage for the poorest sectors of the population. The downside is that around one million people are still not covered by the insurance scheme (Chahed & Arfa, 2014).

In Nigeria, the National Health Insurance Scheme (NHIS) was enacted under Act 35 of 1999 in order to enhance equitable access to healthcare (NHIS, 2000). It was established because of the general poor state of the nation's healthcare services; the excessive dependence and pressure on government provided health facilities; dwindling funding of healthcare in the face of rising cost; and poor integration of private health facilities in the nation's healthcare delivery system (NHIS, 2000).

4.3.1.2   Private (-for-Profit) Health Insurance

In addition to government social insurance schemes, private companies can also play key roles in providing health insurance services. This type is simply called private health insurance (PHI) or private-for-profit health insurance. The private players are in the market to provide quality services, which will enable them to make profit. This type of health insurance is dominant in the capitalist-cum-neoliberal system. Unlike public insurance, where the ultimate goal is to provide health services as a part of welfare service, premiums in PHI are set at a level that provides a profit for third party and provider institutions. Premiums are based on an assessment of the risk of the consumer (or of the group of employees) and the level of benefits provided, rather than as a proportion of the consumer's income (Conn & Walford, 1998).

The essence of this organization is both service and profit maximization. Membership is usually voluntary. In South Africa and some other developing countries, this insurance scheme is widely available, especially in urban areas. In some instances, private insurance schemes operate individual risk-rating. Risk-rating might involve assessment of risk; high-risk individuals (who smoke or have a history of medical complaints) might pay higher premium. There is possibility that low-income, high-risk populations are served mainly by the public sector, while high-income, low-risk populations are generally treated in the private sector (Missoni & Solimano, 2010).

In many African countries, the proportion of contribution of private health insurance (out of total health expenditure) is often relatively low. This probably reflects a number of factors, including high costs and availability of free healthcare in some countries (Witter, 2000). Private health insurance is implemented on a large scale in many countries (including Brazil, Chile, Namibia, Zimbabwe and South Africa) (Spaan et al., 2012). In reality, it has been argued that private health insurance will continue to play only a marginal role in sub-Saharan Africa (Drechsler & Jütting, 2007). The argument of marginal functionality is based on the level socio-economic development. Since there is relatively high level of poverty, non-profit insurance schemes appear to be of critical importance (Drechsler & Jütting, 2007).

4.3.1.3   Community-Based Health Insurance (CBHI) Scheme

Community-Based Health Insurance (CBHI) is a form of private, non-profit health insurance or a form of public insurance meant for the informal sector or lower class. Premiums are not based on assessment of individual risk status. CBHI is "an emerging concept for providing financial protection against the cost of illness and improving access to quality health services for low-income and rural households who are excluded from formal insurance schemes" (Donfouet & Mahieu, 2012). CBIH is usually established through local initiatives with voluntary membership (Wiesmann & Jütting, 2000). When non-governmental organizations or community and development associations provide CBIH, profitmaking is not a central goal. However, adverse selection can be a problem, because CBIH attracts greater numbers of high-risk members (Conn & Walford, 1998). CBHI ensures affordability of healthcare service covered within the scheme. In general, the scheme often covers basic services tailored to the healthcare needs and preferences of the population (Basaza, Pariyo, & Criel, 2009).

Although the premium is usually moderate and the services are often adapted to the specific needs of their clientele, service coverage under CBHI often is not comprehensive. There is always attempt to extend CBHI scheme to cover the rural area that are usually underserved with health services. Individuals in the informal employment are also prioritized; local farmers, petty traders, artisans, lowly-educated and non-literates, and the rural dwellers are usually the major targets of CBHI. The CBHI schemes have been implemented in Benin, Burkina Faso, Cameroon, Côte d'Ivoire, Ghana, Guinea, Kenya, Mali, Nigeria, Senegal, Tanzania, Togo, and Uganda (Basaza et al., 2009; Carrin, Waelkens, & Criel, 2005). In SSA, small community-based schemes and insurance offered through NGOs and other non-profit organizations will have the greatest development potential (Drechsler & Jütting, 2007).

CBHI is a viable means of extending health coverage with financial protection to the community members in low-income countries (Basaza et al., 2009; Donfouet & Mahieu, 2012). It is also simple to set up, although it requires an organized framework. It involves mobilization of adequate and stable resources to sustain the system in a way that will ensure long-term benefits. CBHI is set up, mostly for rural dwellers and the less privileged, to offer financial protection to clients against catastrophic health expenditures. This should ordinarily stimulate more demand for health services, and consequently improve utilization of healthcare services by all socioeconomic groups. CBHI is a major means of promoting social inclusion: it is an effort to cover vulnerable population (without any discrimination) One of the major principles in CBHI is community participation and empowerment. Since CBHI could be developed from community association, it could be a development strategy that ensures that community structures are developed and maintained by community members for a long-term health returns.

4.4   Benefits of Health Insurance

Health insurance is a social security that guarantees the provision of required health service to persons on the payment of nominal contributions at regular intervals. It is a fundamental means of financial protection, which is a major component of UHC. It has also been advocated as a major best practice that can ensure universal health coverage. This is why more and more nations are instituting health insurance schemes in order to meet the healthcare needs of their citizens. A number of benefits of health insurance will be examined.

4.4.1   Financial Protection

Health insurance is a fundamental way of ensuring financial protection against high user fees or out-of-pocket payments. It is essential that households be protected against impoverishment from such expenditures, which may otherwise lead to financial catastrophes for poor households. Spaan et al. (2012) observed that health financing mechanisms were developed to counteract the detrimental effects of user fees, which is a major barrier to healthcare utilization, especially for the marginalized populations. Without financial protection, a poor individual might need to sell his/her property to cover for healthcare costs. Health insurance guarantees that services are provided when needed without instant monetary exchange. In short, health insurance protects families from the financial hardship of huge medical bills.

4.4.2   Improved Healthcare Utilization

Health insurance is a means for improving healthcare utilization (Spaan et al., 2012). A systematic review of US studies shows that there is a positive relationship between health insurance and healthcare utilization and even health outcomes (Freeman, Kadiyalla, Bell, & Martin, 2008). The study specifically reported that health insurance has substantial effects on the use of physician services, preventive services and self-reported health status (Freeman et al., 2008). Health insurance schemes significantly increase the likelihood of utilizing various healthcare services in African countries (Blanchet, Fink, & Osei-Akoto, 2012; Spaan et al., 2012; Woldemichael & Shimeles, 2015). This indicates that if the current health insurance scheme is expanded, more people will benefit from the scheme. Health insurance is therefore an important measure for reaching universal health coverage, which is a major health goal in Africa.

4.4.3 Social Inclusion and Equity in Healthcare

Extending healthcare coverage to all segments of the population is a major challenge in Africa. An ideal health insurance ensures that all population categories, especially the vulnerable, are covered. Various population groups obtain access to healthcare only through health insurance. Since risks are pooled, a wide range of services are equitably available which otherwise might not be the case. Health insurance also ensures equitable distribution of healthcare costs among different income groups. Since most national health insurances are usually compulsory for employees, irrespective of levels of income, this will enhance equitability in health services. The initiation of CBHI also helps to extend healthcare to all community members without discrimination. This is why it has been observed that achieving equitable universal health coverage requires the guarantee of access to essential services, "necessary services for the entire population without imposing an unaffordable burden on individuals or households" (Harris et al., 2011).

4.4.4 Effectiveness of Healthcare System

Health insurance increases the effectiveness of the healthcare system. Effective service is the core of healthcare delivery system. Health insurance ensures payment for health services thereby creating access to health services, which is likely to also improve the quality of health services. For instance, CBHI schemes in Kenya, Uganda and Tanzania were found to improve service quality in health facilities, by increasing essential drug availability and shortening waiting times (Spaan et al., 2012). A secured flow of funds to the health system will likely ensure that the required medicines and technologies are procured to meet clients' needs. In most countries where health insurance is instituted, both the supply and the demand of healthcare increase. The challenge in most African countries is to extend the insurance coverage to the less privileged, rural dwellers and the poor. Apart from equity, this is necessary to enhance the effectiveness of the healthcare system.

4.4.5 Improved Healthcare Funding

Health insurance attracts additional money for health services, above and beyond budgetary allocations from the government. In countries where health insurance has been widely implemented, it is often compulsory. Every individual has the opportunity to register with either the public or private health insurance. Health insurance involves a kind of solidarity contribution from the public, which significantly saves government some fund. Apart from government funding, there is also private investment, the for-profit organizations, and sometimes, non-profit organizations. In general, the majority of consumers are eager to pay for health insurance through taxes rather than (out-of-pocket) payments while they are ill. Health insurance also helps to limit the rise in the costs of healthcare services. Even the rural poor are usually willing to make contribution to a health fund. For instance, studies on willingness to pay for CBHI have found that the rural poor and those in the informal sector are usually willing to enroll in CBHI (Ahmed et al., 2016; Heile, Ololo, & Megersa, 2014).

4.4.6 Improved Health Outcomes

Health insurance generally improves access to healthcare, which is a major predictor of inequalities in health outcomes. Through improved access, health insurance improves health outcomes. Evidence from SSA shows that CBHI expands the use of maternal health services and improves maternal health outcomes (Alison, Peterson, & Hatt, 2013). Most of the studies in SSA target rural populations that are difficult to reach through standard health insurance. CBHI can facilitate availability of advanced care. Health insurance often provides access to maternal services such as C-Section, which otherwise would have been unaffordable to rural dwellers.

4.5 Challenges Militating Against Full Operation of Health Insurance

Despite the laudable benefits of health insurance, there are still a number of challenges affecting its full implementation in Africa. Insurance is a growing market in the developing world, where health problems are highly endemic. In most low-income countries, the state has not been able to fulfill the healthcare needs of the poor, especially of the rural population. While Africa overall has seen some improvement in healthcare funding, it is still inadequate to support many of its healthcare needs. The healthcare situation led to the emergence of many community-based health insurance schemes to improve access to health services and health outcomes (Wiesmann & Jutting, 2001). A popular approach to this problem is mandatory social health insurance, which involves compulsory wage tax deduction to meet health insurance premiums (Gertler and Solon, 2002). National health insurance policy is usually informed by the need to expand the coverage of insurance, but there are often a number of challenges to contend with.

4.5.1 Difficulty in Collecting Revenues

The high cost of insurance administration and the difficulty in controlling payments are crucial issues in low-income countries. This is why the coverage of those in informal employment, rural dwellers and the poor is generally still elusive in many parts of Africa. Available infrastructure is often insufficient to support and manage the payment system and documentation of the citizens. In the informal sector, it is difficult to use wage-based deduction systems. Because the informal economic sector is large, it is difficult to collect revenues, either in the form of taxes or in the form of health insurance contributions (premiums). Moreover, tax collection systems are often inefficient and inequitable (National Academy of Science, 2012). Many of those working in the informal sector are not registered in the national database and their houses not numbered or captured. This lack of population record makes it difficult to administer insurance in many African countries.

4.5.1.1 High Levels of Poverty

The poverty level in Africa is still very high: Considerable proportions of the population are still living below the poverty-line of $1 a day. They may thus be too poor to be able to contribute towards any form of risk pooling of health insurance. And of all the risks facing poor households, health risks—with the resulting catastrophic health expenditures—probably pose the greatest threat to lives and livelihoods (Jutting, 2003). The first challenge is to meet the most essential needs (food, clothing and shelter) before healthcare needs. Where there is still a pressing challenge of meeting the essential needs, contributing to healthcare needs might not be prioritized. Tenkorang (2001) observed that the uncertainty of the timing of illness and unpredictability of its cost make financial provisions for illness difficult for households receiving low and irregular incomes. This leaves the poor more likely to be excluded from insurance because they are too poor to pay and do not have regular employment for meeting regular payments (Gertler and Solon, 2002). This implies that insurance may fail to attract additional fund flow to the health sector where there are high rates of poverty, and where there is limited CBHI.

4.5.1.2 Lopsided Insurance Scheme/Inequality in Insurance Coverage

The problem of urban bias is another major challenge. The distribution of health insurance services tends to be concentrated in urban areas, where the major health facilities are located, and where it is more profitable than in rural areas. This bias is evident in many African countries; hence the gradual introduction of CBHI to cater to the rural areas and the informal sector. Even when the CBHI is instituted, more advanced services might not be accessible in some localities. This signifies that there is still a problem of exclusion from insurance services. In Senegal (for instance) as in most African countries, large proportions of the population are not covered by formal health insurance, and access problems in terms of financing and geographical outreach have been reported (Jutting, 2003).

4.5.1.3 Poor Political Will

Political will is a major ingredient in the initiation and implementation of health insurance schemes. Political will refers to the deliberate planning and efforts of the government to pursue a definite course of action. It requires legislation, budgeting, and judicious utilization of earmarked funds in an efficient manner. It is important for national leaders to recognize the enormous contributions of healthcare in national development and as a core welfare package. Health insurance is a bold step in healthcare financing, and requires deliberate planning by the government to institute or provide a viable atmosphere for insurance stakeholders to operate. The government institutes a majority of the viable insurance schemes in Africa, although the issue of coverage is still a major challenge. Expanding the coverage will require more government financial commitment in order to improve healthcare in Africa.

References

Ahmed, S., Hoque, M. E., Sarker, A. R., Sultana, M., Islam, Z., Gazi, R., Khan, J. A. M. (2016). Willingness-to-pay for community-based health insurance among informal workers in urban Bangladesh. *PLoS One, 11*(2), e0148211. doi:10.1371/journal.pone.0148211.

Alison, B. C., Peterson, L. A., Hatt, L. E. (2013). Effect of health insurance on the use and provision of maternal health services and maternal and neonatal health outcomes: a systematic review. *Journal of Health and Population Nutrition, 31*(4 Suppl 2), S81–S105.

Basaza, R., Pariyo, G., Criel, B. (2009). What are the emerging features of community health insurance schemes in east Africa? *Risk Management and Healthcare Policy, 2*, 47–53.

Blanchet, M. J., Fink, G., Osei-Akoto, I. (2012). The effect of Ghana's national health insurance scheme on healthcare Utilisation. *Ghana Medical Journal, 46*(2), 76–84.

Carrin, G., Waelkens, M., Criel, B. (2005). Community-based health insurance in developing countries: a study of its contribution to the performance of health financing systems. *Tropical Medicine and International Health, 10*(8), 799–811.

Chahed, M. K., & Arfa, C. (2014). Monitoring and evaluating progress towards universal health coverage in Tunisia. *PLoS Medicine, 11*(9), e1001729. doi:10.1371/journal.pmed.1001729.

Conn, C., & Walford, V. (1998). *An introduction to health insurance for low income countries*. DFID, London, Institute for Health Sector Development.

Dickson, D. A., & John, T. S. (1987). *Introduction to insurance*. New York: McGraw Hill.

Donfouet, H. P. P., & Mahieu, P. (2012). Community-based health insurance and social capital: a review. *Health Economics Review, 2*, 5. doi:10.1186/2191-1991-2-5.

Drechsler, D., & Jütting, J. (2007). Different countries, different needs: the role of private health insurance in developing countries. *Journal of Health Politics, Policy and Law, 32*(3), 497–534. doi:10.1215/03616878-2007-012.

Freeman, J. D., Kadiyalla, S., Bell, J. F., Martin, D. P. (2008). The causal effect of health insurance on utilization and outcomes in adults: a systematic review of US studies. *Medical Care, 46*(10), 1023–1032. doi:10.1097/MLR.0b013e318185c913.

Gertler, P., & Solon, O. (2002). Who benefits from social health insurance? Evidence from the Philippines? Unpublished manuscript.

Govender, V., Chersich, M. F., Harris, B., Alaba, O., Ataguba, J. E., Nxumalo, N., Goudge, J. (2013). Moving towards universal coverage in South Africa? Lessons from a voluntary government insurance scheme. *Global Health Action, 6*, 19253. doi:10.3402/gha.v6i0.19253.

Harris, B., Goudge, J., Ataguba, J. E., McIntyre, D., Nxumalo, N., Jikwana, S., Chersich, M. (2011). Inequities in access to healthcare in South Africa. *Journal of Public Health Policy, 32* (Suppl 1), S102–S123.

Heile, M., Ololo, S., Megersa, B. (2014). Willingness to join community-based health insurance among rural households of Debub Bench District, Bench Maji Zone, Southwest Ethiopia. *BMC Public Health, 14*, 591. doi:10.1186/1471-2458-14-591.

Jutting, J. (2003). Health insurance for the poor? Determinant of participation in community-based health insurance scheme in rural Senegal. Technical Paper, Paris, OECD Development Center.

Mehr, R. I., Cammack, E., Rose, T. (1985). *Principles of insurance*. Homewood: Richard D. Irwin, Inc.

Missoni, E., Solimano, G. (2010). Towards universal health coverage: the Chilean experience. World Health Report (2010) Background Paper, No 4.

Naidoo, S. (2012). The South African national health insurance: a revolution in health-care delivery! *Journal of Public Health, 34*(1), 149–150. doi:10.1093/pubmed/fds008.

National Academy of Science (2012). *The continuing epidemiological transition in sub-Saharan Africa: a workshop summary*. Washington: National Academies Press.

National Health Insurance Scheme [NHIS] (2000). *Health insurance handbook*. Abuja: NHIS.

Spaan, E., Mathijssen, J., Tromp, N., McBain, F., ten Have, A., Baltussen, R. (2012). The impact of health insurance in Africa and Asia: a systematic review. *Bulletin of the World Health Organization, 90*, 685–692. doi:10.2471/BLT.12.102301.

Tenkorang, D. A. (2001). Health Insurance for the informal sector in Africa: design features, risk protection and resources mobilisation and risk sharing. Washington, DC: CMH Working Paper Series, No. W. G 3/1.

Wiesmann, D., & Jütting, J. (2000). The emerging movement of community based health insurance in sub-Saharan Africa—experiences and lessons learned. *Afrika Spektrum, 35*, 193–210.

Wiesmann, D., & Jutting, J. (2001). Determinants of health insurance scheme in rural Subsaliava Africa. *Quarterly Journal of International Agriculture, 50*(4), 361–378.

Witter, S. (2000). Health financing in developing and transitional countries. Briefing Paper for Oxfam, G.B.

Woldemichael, A., & Shimeles, A. (2015). Measuring the impact of micro-health insurance on healthcare utilization: a bayesian potential outcomes approach. Working Paper Series No 225 African Development Bank, Abidjan, Côte d'Ivoire.

World Health Organization [WHO] (2013). *The state of health financing in the African region*. Kinshasa, DR Congo: WHO African Region Office.

Chapter 5
African Culture and Health

5.1 Introduction

Culture is universal. Traditions, customs, values and norms are distinct parts of any society. Culture exerts a tremendous influence on all aspects of health, healthcare and health-seeking behaviors and other health-related issues. A major factor influencing health in Africa is culture. It is truly a complex whole with very strong influences on health trajectories and beliefs in Africa. This is why the discourse about health in Africa can never be complete without the cultural discourse. The traditions, customs, values and norms are distinct part of the African people. Culture is, however, not peculiar to Africa; it is universal. Culture gives essence of any person. The starting point of addressing health challenges is to resolve certain culture-related issues which might (scientifically) constitute some determinants of health (see Abubakar et al., 2013; Feyisetan, Asa, & Ebigbola, 1997).

It is a central debate or discourse to ensure adequate cultural considerations in health programs and policies. Or at the basic and general level, to understand the wellbeing of the people: how they behave the way they do and attendant consequences for human health. Culture is everything and everything is immersed in culture. The social organization of the people follows some cultural dictates. Such organization includes power, gender, family, economic and political structures of the people, which invariably affect human health. Specifically, culture has been defined as a complex whole, which includes knowledge, belief, art, law, morals, customs, and any other capabilities and habits acquired by humans as members of society (Tylor, 1871). Most of what individuals learn constituting ways of life is culture. It is acquired throughout lifetime. Whether consciously or unconsciously, humans submit to cultural norms as a member of a society through a gradual reformation of the "uncultured" tendencies.

While over the years, cultural traits have persisted, and serve as fundamental determinant of health in many ramifications; it is still pertinent that the cultural values and beliefs have persisted over time. Some traditional cultural traits have survived modernity. It is often a point to ponder: why traditionalism has survived in the face of modernity? Not only modernity per se, but also strives in the face of scientific explanations. When it comes to conservative African culture and its influences on health, it is not always negative. The rich culture is immersed in ideals that have served positively to elevate the wellbeing of the people. Such traits have been passed from generations to generations while some have actually swept away by modernity. This point about eroding culture is sometimes painful to bear for the conservatives who believe that the African identity is being eroded by modernism. Hence, there have even been some drives to revitalize the African identity and some of its fundamental influences on health. This is because it is believed that cultural traits are somehow functional: they exist because they perform some functions.

Culture is, therefore, a powerful tool, whether in its tangible or intangible form. It shapes all activities of humans and helps in the moral demarcation of right and wrong. Culture is the foundation of ethics. It is the foundation on which other moral and behavioral indicators derive. This is why it is often argued that culture make humans beings, although humans also make cultures. On the influences of culture, one paramount aspect of concern is health. The essence of this chapter is to explore a grand narrative of the African culture in order to draw its implications on health. Before examining such implications, it is important to address the issue of an African culture.

5.2   Is There an African Culture?

Africa is the second largest continent in terms of population. Made up of 54 countries (see Fig. 5.1), it is a multi-ethnic society with over 1000 languages. Every ethnic group has a distinct language and specific cultural traits that are transferred from one generation to the next. Before colonialism and the scramble for Africa, the continent was empire-based. Colonialism ensured some cultural diffusion with the western cultures. Colonialism marked the beginning of industrialization and the incorporation of Africa into the world capitalist system (Amzat & Olutayo, 2009). It marked the beginning of a dual society, with modern and traditional cultures existing side by side. As the continent pushes for modernization, it still recognizes the existence of traditional values. For instance, there is medical pluralism, the existence of both traditional and modern medicine, both of which enjoy considerable patronage.

In terms of regional divisions, the continent has five regions: North Africa, West, Central, East and Southern Africa. In terms of language, most nations have adopted lingua franca (national language[s]) to ensure unification in terms of communication. Anglophone Africa has English as the national language, Arabophone has Arabic, Francophone has French and Lusophone has Portuguese. Some countries recognize more than one language. Despite these divisions, the continent is united into the African Union (AU). North Africa is made up mainly of the Arab region. Sub-

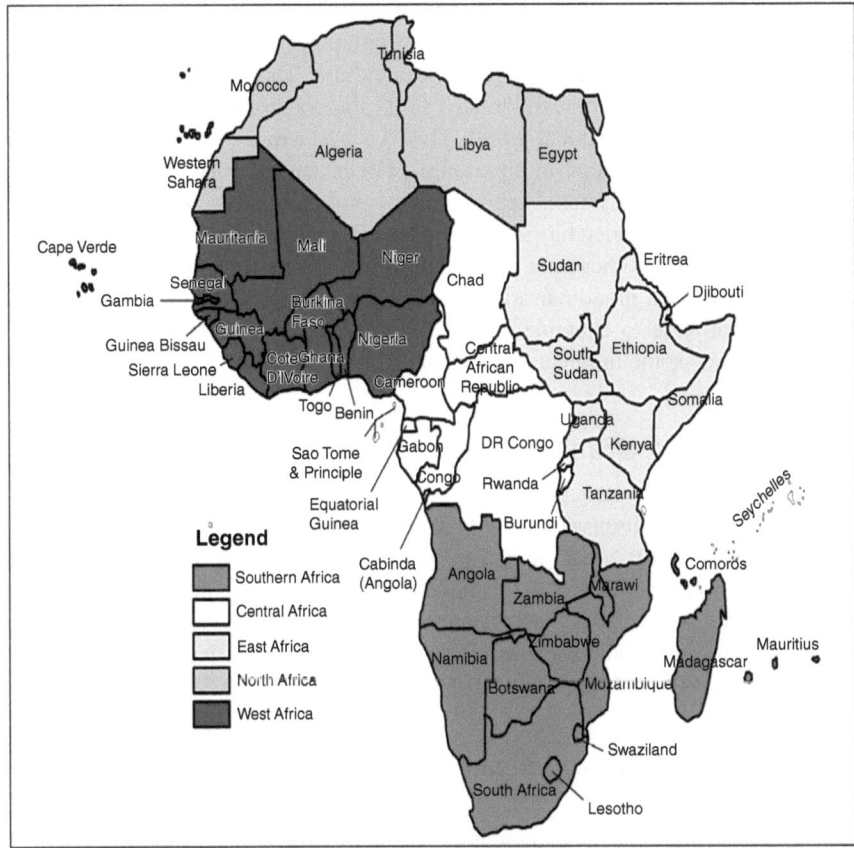

Fig. 5.1 Map of Africa showing countries and regions

Saharan Africa consists of the other four regions (West, Central, East and Southern Africa). The horn of Africa is a peninsula in East Africa containing the countries of Eritrea, Djibouti, Ethiopia and Somalia. It is named after its horn-like shape on the map of Africa and, is a part of SSA (see Fig. 5.1).

Despite the various divergences, Africa shares a linked cultural identity. This is not to deny the diversity, complexity and dynamics of culture across the continent, but an attempt to stress commonalities that point to a possibility of homogeneous African cultural world. Without going deep into other forms of divisions, the critical question is whether there is an African culture. The aforementioned issues signify that Africa is not a country but a continent of diverse people with different traditions. Even within every country, there are diverse traditional cultures. In Ethiopia, Sudan, Tanzania, Nigeria, Kenya and South Africa for instance, there are hundreds of ethnic groups speaking different languages. This multiethnic situation is reflected in most African countries. This is why sometimes there are inter-ethnic conflicts.

The chapter focuses on African culture and health. The foundational argument is that despite these social variations and geographical divisions, there are grand similarities, which can be merged as African culture. This implies that certain cultural denominations can be extrapolated to all the countries. This is not only true for Africa, even for the global world. This is why there are cultural universals, a kind of traits that are found in all cultures. For instance, every culture has a language, has age grade system, gender norms, dressing codes, morals (specifying wrongs and rights), leadership structure, marriage patterns and so on. While there are variations in how these are prosecuted, they represent significant commonalities based on which grand narratives can be developed. The section will dwell on this grand narrative to examine some relevant common themes from cultures in Africa and draw some implications for health.

5.3   Towards a Grand Narrative of African Culture and Health

From the foregoing discussion, this is simply an eagle-eye approach to provide a general overview. By grand narrative, it simply means exploiting the common grounds to generalize. This is not to undermine some specific micro circumstances or to underplay some observable differences across African communities. Following this macroanalytic approach, some common features of African culture will be explained in relation to health.

5.3.1   Communitarianism and Social Capital

One common feature of African culture is the strong social bond. This is what classical sociologists, Ferdinand Tonnies called *Gemeinschaft*, and Emile Durkheim referred to it as mechanical solidarity. Communitarianism here is described as a form of cultural practice, which emphasizes the responsibility of the individual to the community and the social importance of community life instead of individual life. It is a practice of collectivism, where group feelings and responsibility supersedes individual feeling. Social bond implies a high sense of social support, extended familial bonding and communal relations. Mechanical solidarity is characterized with low levels of individualism and high levels of collectivism. It is a society that is fraught with collective conscience, responsible for high level of cooperation in the society. This social cohesion is evident among individuals in African society. In general, this is a source of cooperation within any group. The Yoruba community in Nigeria is a mechanical solidarity community, as are the Maasai of Kenya and Tanzania, the Hausa in West Africa and the Zulu of southern Africa. The modern culture is characterized by organic solidarity, which is premised on individualism. While African society is modernizing, this sense of collectivism has survived all forms of social alteration that Africa has encountered.

Collective conscience informs the availability of a vital resource called social capital. Reciprocal support and assistance are part of the bedrock of the extended family and communal relationships in African societies. Social capital can be viewed as "social resources," signifying the links and support that individuals can access at a particular time as a member of a group (Amzat & Razum, 2014). Social capital signifies the good-will, fellowship, mutual sympathy and social intercourse among a group of individuals. This is a vital resource among various African groups. What often exists are bonding ties within homogenous groups, i.e., strong ties that connect family members, neighbors, and close friends and colleagues (Islam, Merlo, Kawachi, Lindstrom, & Gerdtham, 2006). These ties have been identified as major determinants of health (Carpiano, 2006, 2007; Kawachi, 2006). In the African context, where social safety nets are inadequate, many families rely on a network of reciprocal assistance provided by members of a larger group: the men support the women or vice versa, the young support the aged, and the employed support the unemployed (Amzat & Razum, 2014). The effects of social capital on health are larger in African societies because of the general low level of development. There is reliance on network ties and mutual fellowship.

Despite dire conditions in Africa—of high poverty, inadequate health services and high disease burden—one major buffer is the high level of social capital derived from associational life. This implies that community life is a major shield from some of the worst effects of deprivation. For instance, informal healthcare and support can be provided in case of illness, and "… hospital bills might be contributed; baby-sitting assistance can be provided; and cooking, washing and other supportive care might be provided by other family or community members" (Amzat & Razum, 2014, p. 101). Social capital and cooperative life signal a useful framework for what constitutes health-supporting environments and buffer points, in terms of needs (Eriksson, 2011). It is further noted that mapping and mobilization of social capital in local communities may be one way of achieving community action for health promotion (Eriksson, 2011). The intergenerational support in society in the absence of functional social security (e.g., pension schemes) is a vital indicator of social capital in Africa.

Other vital cultural implications on health in term of community life are as follows:

1. Culture dictates level of social capital in the society, and in case of illness, the level of social support from community members. As it has been pointed out, this can help to stimulate a sense of belonging, and in African settings, in many cases, material support might be provided.
2. Culture contributes to the level of social needs and the intensity of fulfillment of such needs. Social needs are not quantifiable and serve as vitalizing measures, which also sustain human wellbeing/health. For instance, such social needs are particularly important for quality of life of the aged.

5.3.2   Sociocultural Dualism

Africa is a dual (or pluralistic) society, with characterized by worldviews that are sometimes at odds with one another. Dualism in this regard implies a number of issues. The meaning of sociocultural dualism in this respect is not constrained to the economic realm, but extends to a more divergent social context. Sociocultural dualism is the clashing of an imported social system with an indigenous social system of another style (Boeke, 1953). In this case, it is not about clashing but co-existence of two traditions. This is a mix of both imported and local traditions—of modernism and traditionalism—both prevailing with certain levels of sophistication, although usually with a gradual movement towards modernism. This implies that modernism has not completely assimilated traditionalism. The debate is still ongoing as to whether there was an interruption of a developing traditional system, which would have taken a different course, perhaps better off, than the incorporation into a new system called modernism.

First, the different worldviews, both (indigenous) traditional and modern, are pervasive in every setting. Traditional conservatism and progressive modernism exist side-by-side, sometimes in a competing stance and sometimes complementary. More and more, the relevant forms of dualistic fission run along the line of rural/urban sectors and traditional/modern sectors and formal/informal sectors (Singer, 1970). This dualism also applies to traditional medicine versus modern medicine. The tendency for technological developments to produce internal dualism in under-developed countries is always a possibility because some conservative ideas, traditions and practices will survive for considerable time.

A typical African country is both urban and rural. The urban centers are characterized by modern amenities, while the rural areas are usually short of such amenities. The rural areas mostly rely on traditional methods/measures. For instance, African rural societies are generally underserved with modern healthcare facilities, so that they mostly depend upon traditional medicine for their healthcare. In most parts of Africa, there is still a strong belief in supernatural and mystical causes of diseases, while at the same time some biomedical ideas still prevail—both conflicting and complementary at the same time. There is the possibility of a combined therapy from both traditions (modern and traditional medicine). Dualism extends to the co-existence of both a formal health sector and a high prevalence of home treatment and other related informal or undocumented health services. For instance, buying drugs from drug stores without a (formal) prescription is common. And use of traditional medicine is very common, despite that in many countries there are no proper guidelines to regulate the informal sector.

5.3.3   Traditional Notions and Practices

Beyond the dual existence of traditional and modern sectors, traditional notions and practices are crucial aspect of the African culture. This is often observed in the conception of health and response to disease including practices that hold implications for human health. A traditional notion signifies a general understanding, definable or not, or sometimes imperfect—a general conception or idea of social events within an ethnic group. It is a general perception of events. On the other hand, traditional practices are manifestation of culture through distinct customary actions developed over a period of time. Customary rites are part of practices, and influenced how notions are developed and sustained within a culture. Some of those notions and practices have to do with health or influence health. African culture is imbued with distinct traditional notions and practices.

In terms of health, traditional notions are close to what is regarded as lay conception of health. The traditional context has been a central subject in the understanding of African health. There are notions regarding disease causality, treatment patterns and outcomes. Notions relate to belief regarding disease realities and symptom evaluation. Culture gives meaning to disease, helps in defining somatic and behavioral indications to sickness (Bode, 2011). "Culture does not work in a mechanic and deterministic way, but provides people with more than one way in which somatic and behavioral dysfunctions can be converted into socially recognized sicknesses" (Bode, 2011). Such cultural function is termed here as traditional notions.

There are also significant traditional practices; some enhance health while some aggravate disease vulnerability. This is why some practices are termed as harmful traditional practices because they have deleterious effects on human health. The harmful practices include female genital cutting (FGC); forced feeding of women; early marriage; facial scarification, widowhood rites, son preference, wife battery and other forms of discriminatory practices. Such notions are dynamic. Some of these traditional notions are shaped by education, health literacy, and general level of development. With time, they can be modified through behavioral change and other health-related programs. There is gradual international recognition of the harmful practices as root causes of the relative care for women and eventual health consequences. It is also important to encourage certain traditional notions, which are not detrimental to disease control efforts.

It is important to reiterate some important points. Therefore, summarily:

1. Culture informs perceptions of health/disease, especially in terms of causality. The cultural indication of etiology provides useful measure of understanding lay conception of health i.e., how people make sense of the causes of the symptom and how to respond to it. In many cases, there are subjective dimensions, which affect health and illness behavior.
2. Culture is embedded in some traditional practices, some of which hold implications for human health. As earlier mentioned, some practices are harmful to human health by reinforcing vulnerability or discriminatory practices (such as gender discrimination and stigmatization).
3. Culturally-constructed concepts of health and disease are powerful tools in health information and communication. Concepts are designated to describe and understand disease condition in day-to-day communication. For instance, what is the cultural designate of HIV? How can the concept be used to promote understanding of the disease and enhance its control?
4. Traditional cultural notions might depict some misconceptions. In many instances, such notions deviate from biomedical notions. For instance, the perception of witchcraft as the cause of a child's death is common in Africa, even

when the death is actually due to malaria (see Jegede, 2002; Sabuni, 2007). In some instances, people are fatalistic about child mortality, viewing it as the will of God. In such instances, misconception must be addressed to enhance disease understanding and also enhance control efforts.

5. Culture also helps individuals make sense of illness experience. It helps in the interpretation of bodily indication, and specifies care-seeking options (see Kleinman, 2013). Apart from experience, expression of pain or symptom is also mediated by culture. Some cultures favor concealment of pain and discomfort. Where a culture of modesty is strict, discussion of sensitive issues such as sexual and reproductive problems are not usually openly expressed.

6. Culture influences health-related preferences. For instance, gender concordance (of the patient and provider) is strongly advocated in some cultures. The preference may extend to patterns of treatment. In some societies, drugs with alcoholic content are often preferred as the last resort. Such variations in preference may extend to different aspects of healthcare and spell important considerations for population health.

5.3.4   Religiosity

Africa is a religious continent—this is why religion is a sensitive issue in Africa. Religion is a unified form of belief. The most common religions in Africa include Christianity, Islam and traditional religions. For each of them, there are a number of denominations. African people take religion as a major aspect of their way of life with various level of intensity. People are prayerful and engage in many kinds of rituals. It is a common practice for people to invoke some ritual rites in connection with health. There are a number of ways that religion affects health. Religious prescriptions do have implication for health. For instance, religion helps in regulating sexuality. The major denominations of Islam and Christianity forbid pre-marital sex, extra-marital relationship, abortion and so on. While there are prescriptions, conformity is another issue. The high rate of multiple sexual partnerships as a risk factor in HIV might signal that conformity with sexual modesty (in religious terms) is sometimes compromised. For the adherents of a particular faith which forbids alcohol, that could help to reduce alcohol-related diseases.

People also hold belief in the roles of God or gods in human health. It is often believed that God is protective and could give healing to any form of ailment. This might be the basis of prayers for protection against all forms of evils responsible for ill-health, and also for recuperation. Within religions contexts, it is also believed that some evil forces can inflict people with some forms of illness. Therefore, adherents need to also pray in order to avert the occurrence of illness. In some extreme cases, some believe in the power of prayers without resorting to modern medicine for help. Fasting, alms giving, and other religious acts are common to seek the mercy of God against all forms of illness.

Some traditional practices such as early marriage and polygyny are usually rationalized with some religious reasons in Muslim-dominated Africa countries. Use of contraceptives and family size preference are also shaped by religion. For instance, some religious denominations reject certain contraceptives except natural ones (such as the withdrawal method and abstinence). A study in Nigeria observed that there is sufficient evidence that religious beliefs have an influence on contraceptive use in Nigeria, as Christians are more likely to use contraception than Muslims (Osuafor & Mturi, 2013). That is why it has been observed that one of the major challenges to improving family planning coverage in Africa is the existence of many conflicting cultural and religious beliefs. It is often the case for many adherents to follow the prescriptions of their congregation leaders. Therefore, engaging faith leaders might also be a good strategy in changing peoples' opinion/behavior about health-related issues.

In general, religion is part of personal identity and could inform how healthcare is accessed. It is possible to ask for some procedures mainly for religious reason. Circumcision of male children among the Muslims is a typical example. While many western nations do not conduct male circumcisions, predominantly Muslim nations still practice this as a religious rite. It is possible to reject some procedures for religious reason, such as Jehovah's Witnesses refusing blood transfusions. It is also common for some religious organizations to support the provision of healthcare. The bottom-line is that religion is a major institution that shapes every aspect of human life. It is a force dominating individuals in Africa. Congregations are usually full of people praying for protection (i.e., against calamities), and prosperity (to escape poverty and related socio-economic calamities).

It is important to reiterate some important points. Therefore, summarily:

1. Religious teachings often influence beliefs about the origins and nature of disease. For instance, in religious circles, some diseases are regarded as a result of sins or religious infringements. In Islam and Christianity, condom is still perceived as a symbol of immorality outside marriage. Therefore, condom is not a preached option in HIV control among many religious adherents.
2. Religion also influences care-seeking options. For instance, diseases often require pleasing of the God through repentance, fasting and prayers. There is high prevalence of healing through deliverance/casting of demons. The faith-based healers contribute to healthcare provision in Africa.
3. Religion also enhances positive psychological state (see Oman & Thoresen, 2002). It helps to stimulate immunity both in terms of health and illness. It helps people to pull themselves together in the face of challenges through hope, faith and inner peace. The strong belief in prayers and other atonement process could positively function to ensure well-being (like placebo effects [because the actual process of influence cannot be scientifically established]).
4. Religion helps to influence risk behaviors through series of prescriptions and proscriptions. For instance, some religious denominations curtail some risk behaviour including some sexual behaviors, smoking, dietary behaviours, and alcohol consumption (see also Amzat & Razum, 2014).

5.3.5 Gender Inequality

Classification or ranking of people based on class, age, status and gender is also a major feature of African culture. Stratification can be based on achievement (achieved status) and ascription (ascribed status). Achieved status includes socio-economic indicators such as income, education and occupation while ascribed status is based on characteristics that an individual cannot control, such as age and gender. Stratification is how humans organize themselves into various cultural and social groupings with some form of ranking. A social stratum is a group of individuals who share a similar social characteristic. Social stratification is very evident in African culture. It is usually a form of inequality system and some extend to discriminatory practices. Existence of social hierarchies cut across all cultures but there are variations in social gaps: in some, the gap is very wide. Such stratification has implications for health. African culture is still a culture of gender inequality, age, grade and class system. The focus here is on gender.

Africa is a gendered society. Gender is a social creation, involving differentiation of social roles and unequal power relations between the sexes. While most societies are gendered, the gender gap is still very wide in Africa. While gender issues concern both men and women, the focus here will be on women because they bear the brunt of gender inequality in African society. Amzat and Grandi (2011, p. 140) made some important points regarding the gender framework: First, women are vulnerable in the in the context of relationships. They are not treated as equal to men. This inequality can go from conception to death; second, women often face oppression within gender relations as their autonomy is usually threatened. Women often have to conform to patriarchal norms; third, women often face discrimination and violence. Gender-based violence is a major issue in Africa. And fourth, resource allocation is often unfavorable to women. Access to paid employment is limited, and poverty is higher among women. Women's access to resources and its affordability are often threatened. In many instances, women are dependent on male partners for required resources.

Gender is a fundamental determinant of health in Africa. MacPherson, Richards, Namakhoma, and Theobald (2014) observed that gender inequality is a factor influencing many health issues among women including sexual and reproductive health, maternal health and HIV in Eastern and Southern Africa. It is further observed that the health systems significantly disadvantage women in terms of access to care. Chirowa, Atwood, and Putten (2013) confirmed that countries with high gender inequality captured by the gender inequality index were associated with high maternal mortality ratios, compared to countries with lower gender inequality. Sociocultural practices and norms and economic factors put females at a disadvantage and relatively higher risk of being infected with HIV compared to men (Abubakar & Kitsao-Wekulo, 2015). Other determinants of health such as education, income and occupation also exhibit gender dimensions—all of which unfavorable to women. Therefore, a consideration of health and healthcare in Africa must integrate gender considerations in such a way as to alleviate the inequity faced by women.

5.3.6 Power Distance

Another major important consideration in African culture is power distance. Hofstede (2001) identified power distance as a dimension of culture. Power distance is a form of power relations signifying the gap in power between the upper and lower strata, which is culturally entrenched. The point is whether the gap is wide or not. This is a kind of social hierarchy. Apart from gender, there are other social hierarchies within African context. In terms of age grade, there is hierarchy according to age between the young and the old. In general, those with relatively high status enjoy certain privileges in the society far better than the people with low status. This power distance is still very large in Africa between the old and the young, the rich and the poor, the health professionals and patients. Social distance still remains existential issue well entrenched in the social system and conformity to the hierarchy norms is expected at all times. The socially underprivileged are the voiceless, and incidentally, the most vulnerable.

In many African countries, the youth are still not visible in the political space. This accounts for reduced public participation of the youth. Intergenerational dialogue is often difficult as the young must respect the elders and there is cultural shyness preventing communication between the generations. This is one of the reasons why parent-child communication on sensitive matters (such as sexual health and rights) is not common (Muhammad & Mamdouh, 2012). The notion of subordination is still prevalent. It should be noted that all forms of inequality are usually detrimental to health and healthcare. There is also power gap between the professional and the patient. The patients are often regarded as subordinate and have to comply with the physicians' instructions. This is why there is persistent paternalism in healthcare. Most times, patients' rights and desires are less considered in the health system. The physician is usually autocratic. It is not uncommon for healthcare providers not to inform patients about diagnosis, risks, benefits, and their right to refusal.

5.4 Culture and Health: A Concise Note to the Health Practitioners

Culture impacts health. Health practitioners need to be aware of the deep cultural imprints among certain groups that can create additional challenges for healthcare professionals (including public health professionals). This is why cultural competence is key, as it provides overall excellence in healthcare and health system (Ihara, 2004). Cultural competence in healthcare "is defined as the ability of providers and organizations to effectively deliver healthcare services that meet the social, cultural, and linguistic needs of patients" (Betancourt, Green, & Carrillo, 2002; Ihara, 2004). This is why some social science training is relevant to healthcare professionals. Healthcare itself is carried out in a relational context between the clients and the professionals. Healthcare should be mediated by both professional ethics and cultural values. The professionals need to understand lay perceptions of health in order to grasp some cultural understanding and barriers to effective treatment plan.

It is important to be sensitive to certain cultural trajectories. Such sensitivity can promote trust and acceptance of healthcare, and consequently better healthcare. By implication, it is important to provide training to increase cultural awareness, knowledge, and skills (Ihara, 2004). Public health practitioners also need to have deep cultural understandings in developing health interventions that will respect cultural issues without reinforcing any tradition of inequality or discrimination. Healthcare professionals need to de-emphasize health-related cultural bias (such as gender inequality) against some segments of the society. In order to understand health information, culture-specific attitudes and values should be incorporated into health promotion tools (Ihara, 2004). For instance, graphics in health promotion tool should conform to general cultural standards.

References

Abubakar, A., & Kitsao-Wekulo, P. (2015). Gender and health inequalities in sub-Saharan Africa: the case of HIV. In S. Safdar & N. Kosakowska-Berezecka (Eds), *Psychology of gender through the lens of culture* (pp. 395–408). Cham, Switzerland: Springer International Publishing.

Abubakar, A., Van Baar, A., Fischer, R., Bomu, G., Gona, J. K., Newton, C. R. (2013). Sociocultural determinants of health-seeking behaviour on the Kenyan coast: a qualitative study. *PLoS One, 8*(11), e71998. doi:10.1371/journal.pone.0071998.

Amzat, J., & Grandi, G. (2011). Gender context of personalism in bioethics. *Developing World Bioethics, 11*(3), 136–145.

Amzat, J., & Olutayo, O. A. (2009). Nigeria, capitalism and the question of equity. *The Anthropologist, 11*(4), 239–246.

Amzat, J., & Razum, O. (2014). *Medical Sociology in Africa*. Cham, Switzerland: Springer International Publishing.

Betancourt, J. R., Green, A. R., Carrillo, J. E. (2002). *Cultural competence in healthcare: emerging frameworks and practical approaches*. New York: The Commonwealth Fund.

Bode, M. (2011). The transformations of disease in expert and lay medical cultures. *Journal of Ayurveda and Integrative Medicine, 2*(1), 14–20.

Boeke, J. H. (1953). *Economics and economic policy of dual societies*. New York: International Secretariat, Institute of Pacific Relations.

Carpiano, R. M. (2006). Toward a neighborhood resource-based theory of social capital for health: can Bourdieu and sociology help? *Social Science and Medicine, 62*, 165–175.

Carpiano, R. M. (2007). Neighborhood social capital and adult health: an empirical test of a Bourdieu-based model. *Health and Place, 13*(3), 639–655.

Chirowa, F., Atwood, S., Putten, M. (2013). Gender inequality, health expenditure and maternal mortality in sub-Saharan Africa: a secondary data analysis. *African Journal of Primary Health Care and Family Medicine, 5*(1), 471, 5 pages. doi:10.4102/phcfm.v5i1.471.

Eriksson, M. (2011). Social capital and health—implications for health promotion. *Global Health Action, 4*, doi:10.3402/gha.v4i0.5611.

Feyisetan, B. J., Asa, S., Ebigbola, J. A. (1997). Mothers' management of childhood diseases in Yorubaland: the influence of cultural beliefs. *Health Transition Review, 7*, 221–234.

Hofstede, G. (2001). *Culture's consequences: comparing values, behaviors, institutions, and organizations across nations*. 2nd ed. Thousand Oaks: Sage Publications.

Ihara, E. (2004). Cultural competence in health care: is it important for people with chronic conditions? Georgetown Health Policy Institute, Issue Brief Number 5. https://hpi.georgetown. edu/agingsociety/pubhtml/cultural/cultural.html. Accessed 11 June 2016.

Islam, M. K., Merlo, J., Kawachi, I., Lindstrom, M., Gerdtham, U.-G. (2006). Social capital and health: does egalitarianism matter? A literature review. *International Journal of Equity in Health, 5*(1), 3.

Jegede, A. S. (2002). The Yoruba cultural construction of health and illness. *Nordic Journal of African Studies, 11*(3), 322–335.

Kawachi, I. (2006). Commentary: social capital and health—making the connections one step at a time. *International Journal of Epidemiology, 35*(4), 989–993.

Kleinman, A. (2013). From illness as culture to caregiving as moral experience. *New England Journal of Medicine, 368*, 1376–1377.

MacPherson, E. E., Richards, E., Namakhoma, I., Theobald, S. (2014). Gender equity and sexual and reproductive health in Eastern and Southern Africa: a critical overview of the literature. *Glob Health Action, 7*, doi:10.3402/gha.v7.23717.

Muhammad, Y. Y., & Mamdouh H. M. (2012). Mother-daughter communication about sexual and reproductive health in rural areas of Alexandria, Egypt. Mena Working Paper Series Population Reference Bureau. http://www.prb.org/pdf12/mother-daughter-mena-workingpaper. pdf. Accessed 13 June 2016.

Oman, D., & Thoresen, C. E. (2002). 'Does religion cause health?': differing interpretations and diverse meanings. *Journal of Health Psychology, 7*(4), 365–380.

Osuafor, G. N., & Mturi, A. J. (2013). Do religious beliefs influence use of contraception among currently married women in Nigeria? *Journal of Social Development in Africa, 28*(1), 187–212.

Sabuni, P. L. (2007). Dilemma with the local perception of causes of illnesses in Central Africa: muted concept but prevalent in everyday life. *Qualitative Health Research, 17*, 1280–1291. doi:10.1177/1049732307307864.

Singer, H. W. (1970). Dualism revisited: a new approach to the problems of the dual society in developing countries. *Journal of Developing Societies, 7*(1), 60–75.

Tylor, E. B. (1871). *Primitive culture: researches into the development of mythology, philosophy, religion, art, and custom Volume 1*, London: John Murray.

Chapter 6
Traditional Medicine in Africa

6.1 Introduction

Traditional medicine (TM) is still highly relevant to healthcare in Africa. WHO observed that up to 80% of African population still use TM, especially for their primary health needs. Even in developed countries, it is gaining in popularity; more than 40% of people in many countries including Australia, Canada, USA, Belgium and France have used alternative medicine (which included TM) (WHO, 2002). The extent of use is true considering the arrays of practitioners and their availability across African communities and the scarcity of modern healthcare services (in terms of availability and affordability). It should, however, be noted that modern healthcare occupies the frontline in healthcare delivery in Africa. Major efforts of African government are usually channeled towards improving modern healthcare. However, a number of African countries have recognized TM as an alternative care system that can contribute to alleviating the disease burden in Africa. Although there has not been enough research into TM to actually measure the extent of this contribution, most works on health-seeking behaviors have always highlighted the relevance and use of traditional medicine in Africa (see Atwine, Hultsjo, Albin, & Hjelm, 2015; Cunnama & Honda, 2016; Stanifer et al., 2015). Therefore, the contribution of TM in healthcare delivery in Africa is still under discussion.

As it will later be explained, TM was the major means of healthcare during the pre-colonial Africa. It has always been part of the culture of care and incidentally has survived several thousands of years in meeting the healthcare needs of the population. Sometimes, there is a tension between tradition and modern medicine. Modern medicine has brought new ways of caring for the sick through series of scientific breakthroughs, while TM is striving on experience and traditional knowledge. The essence of this chapter is not to compare the two medical traditions, but it should be noted that they operate on two different worldviews (see Amzat & Razum, 2014). This is why it has been observed that there is a kind of medical pluralism in Africa (like everywhere else, anyway). This medical pluralism is about the co-existence of

© Springer International Publishing AG 2018
J. Amzat, O. Razum, *Towards a Sociology of Health Discourse in Africa*,
DOI 10.1007/978-3-319-61672-8_6

modern and traditional medicine. The co-existence tends to competition, conflict and complementarity (3Cs). Competition often occurs in terms of claims of relevance, and even sometimes superiority, from TM practitioners.

The main drive in many African countries is towards integrating TM with modern medicine—in a way that it complements the efforts of modern healthcare practitioners. This sometimes causes for conflict, since one is from the biomedical sciences and the other from traditional knowledge. Irrespective of the prevailing concerns, TM is part of an established health discourse in Africa. This chapter will introduce readers to the major issues around TM as a complementary or alternative form of healthcare in Africa. The chapter progresses with the meaning of traditional medicine, the historical and current overview of TM in Africa and the relevance and challenges of traditional medicine in Africa. Throughout this chapter, "traditional medicine" refers to complementary or alternative medicine or non-conventional medicine, while "modern medicine" refers to conventional or allopathic medicine, which is the dominant healthcare scheme in Africa.

6.2   What is Traditional Medicine?

Traditional medicine (sometimes called ethno-medicine, native or folk medicine) is not unique to Africa, as it can be obtained in other continents as well. Most TM is culture-specific, as it is not universally similar across cultures. This is why there are African TM, Chinese TM, and so on. Even within Africa, there are a number of variations from country to country and culture to culture. In general, traditional medicine is the "sum total of the knowledge, skills, and practices based on the theories, beliefs, and experiences indigenous to different cultures, whether explicable or not, used in the maintenance of health as well as in the prevention, diagnosis, improvement or treatment of physical and mental illness" (WHO, 2002, 2013). It includes the use of plants, animals, and minerals in medicinal preparation, spiritual therapies, manual techniques and exercises applied to maintain social, physical and mental wellbeing. TM includes sophisticated systems such as acupuncture, ayurvedic medicine, Arabic unani medicine, and other techniques.

In general, TM has distinct features (see Amzat & Razum, 2014). First, it is based on a traditional/cultural worldview, hence the culture-specific versions of TM. The cultural history dictates the direction and use of traditional medicine. Not all traditional medicine can be applied across cultures, because the spiritual processes are often distinct based on an individual's culture and worldview. People identify with traditional medicine because it conforms to their collective consciousness and ancestral origin.

Second, traditional medicine involves a spiritual aspect, which is highly diabolical. This is why WHO (2002) observed that, it may be highly secretive, mystical and extremely localized. This is the aspect often not explicable in biomedical term. It is often passed orally from one generation to the next. It is often difficult to find any comprehensive literature on the practical aspect of traditional medicine, especially the spiritual aspect. The incantations, the invocations of the gods and the rituals are the core aspects. This mysticism makes TM less amenable to scientific testing.

Third, there is a physical aspect, which can be amenable to science. The physical aspect often includes the minerals, plants and animals and other physical components, which scientists recognize as containing potent ingredients that can treat diseases. Traditional healers are known for herbal preparations made from raw or processed plants (leaves, bark, roots, etc.). They sometimes also prepare concoctions and lotions with the use of both plant and animal parts.

Fourth, TM substantially relies on experience rather than experiment. This is why most of their claims cannot be scientifically substantiated. The experiences in the use of different substances have been with the practitioners over the years, and can always make recommendations from experiential knowledge. The experience is passed from one generation to the other, mostly in informal manners. And those who have the experience, through informal attachment or apprenticeship to a known healer (for learning or familial line) are usually recognized as healers in the community.

A traditional healer is a person recognized in the community as knowledgeable in the use of plants and animals and other mineral substances based on the relevant socio-cultural and religious backgrounds, in the prevention, diagnosis and treatment of diseases, infirmities and maintenance of social wellbeing (WHO, 2002). Community recognition is key in the practice of traditional medicine, as there is no formal entry based on formal training or qualification. The healers are mostly residents of the community they serve, found both in urban and rural areas (more in the latter), and relate to personal and social histories to adjudicate with the gods and other supernatural forces that might explain physical, psychological, and social condition. Beyond the treatment of ill-health, the traditional healers are also relevant in resolving personal issues, this is why social issues or wellbeing feature as one of their major responsibilities.

One major factor responsible for the continuous relevance of the traditional medical practitioner is the holistic or totalistic approach. It takes account of the holistic interconnectedness of physical body, mind, spirit, ancestral antecedence and social relations connected to human wellbeing. This explains why they also find remedies for personal and social issues such as unemployment, economic insecurity/poverty, marriage instability and personal protection (against enemies and evil forces) among others. With the high rate of socio-personal problems, the healers attract high patronage from various people seeking solutions to such problems. While some readers might want to raise some questions regarding traditional medicinal mediation in socio-personal problems, as previously mentioned, the essence here is not to dabble into the claims of the traditional healers but to examine some of their activities and relevance regarding population wellbeing.

Traditional medical practitioners in Africa have developed some specializations over the years. Amzat and Razum (2014) identified a number of specializations, including:

1. **Herbalists**: these are individuals who are highly knowledgeable in the use of herbal mixtures to diagnose, prevent and treat medical conditions. They are usually the most visible specialization of TM. The specialization is a kind of traditional herbalism. The herbalists use medicinal plants and animal parts.

2. **Diviners**: these are highly "technical" experts of TM. The diviners normally have enormous spiritual powers to see beyond the ordinary. They are believed to have inner eyes to observe supernatural and mystical forces that might account for a medical or social ailment. The diviners have mediumistic powers to mediate with the gods or ancestors. The major rituals, sacrifices, and spiritual invocation are in the domain of the diviners.

3. **Traditional bonesetters**: this category specializes in traditional orthopedic practice. They mostly do fracture repairs. Some of them use splints and bamboo stick or rattan cane or palm leaf axis with cotton thread or cloth wrapped tightly around the injury before applying herbs and other spiritual means (Dada, Yunusa, & Giwa, 2011).

4. **Traditional Birth Attendants (TBAs)**: The TBAs also called traditional or lay midwives. Apart from the herbalists, this category is also very visible because they offer essential care relating to child and maternal health. They are predominantly women who attend to mothers during childbirth and also care for newborns.

5. **Faith-based Healers**: because of the high level of religiosity in Africa, this category is also popular and widely used. They are religious people who use spiritual healing processes that including prayers and fasting. They are Christian and Islamic clerics who perform all sorts of deliverance and healing by appealing to divine intervention. Faith healers are particularly important because they are believed to offer protection from witchcraft and evil forces, which make people ill.

6. **Traditional Psychiatrists**: Traditional healing is also available to those with all forms of mental/psychological issues. Traditional psychiatrists focus on mental aspects of wellbeing. Psychological issues are often attributed to supernatural and mystical forces; hence, traditional healers are often consulted for treatment.

7. **Traditional Surgeons**: Itinerant traditional surgeons are also available to perform many procedures, including tooth extraction, incising and draining abscesses, uvulectomy, circumcision, piercing, facial tribal marks, inguinal hernia surgery, non-invasive cataract luxation and surgery on closed and open fractures (Miles & Ololo, 2003, p. 505).

6.3   Traditional Medicine in Africa: Some Historical Notes and Relevance

The history of healthcare is as old as the history of man. Maintenance of wellbeing is an imperative aspect of life. It is needless to say that what is called traditional medicine was historically the mainstay of healthcare in precolonial Africa. It is simply developed based on the imperativeness of care. Whether in Europe or America, all forms of medicine started with native medicine. The transformation from native to modern is historical—a history of development in knowledge leading to refinement of practices. Sometimes, the refinement is simply called modernization aided through scientific revolution. All forms of medicine still significantly rely on the same raw materials: minerals, plants and animals. The use of medicinal plants, minerals and other natural products is a fundamental element of the African traditional healthcare system (and elsewhere) and is regarded as the oldest and the most assorted of all therapeutic systems (including modern medicine) (Mahomoodally, 2013). But modern medicine has progressed significantly in evidence-based approach, precision, logic and standardization. This is why TM is often considered healthcare based on experience rather than on experimentation. It is not completely correct to claim that TM is not at all evidence-based. From scientific point of view, the spiritual aspect cannot be empirically tested, while the physical aspect can.

Abdullahi (2011) observed that TM is the oldest form of healthcare that has survived the test of time especially because of its continuous relevance in the maintenance of human wellbeing. It is further observed that it is an ancient and culture-bound method of healing that humans have used to cope with various diseases that have threatened their existence and survival from pre-modern times to the present. Similarly, TM is a socio-cultural heritage, which was wrongly challenged as primitive by the colonialists, and unreligious by the missionaries, and barbaric by conventional medical practitioners (Elujoba, Odeleye, & Ogunyemi, 2005). The historical antecedents are similar in other continents; TM is a result of historical circumstances and cultural beliefs (Romero-Daza, 2002; WHO, 2002).

As previously observed, modern medicine has grown out of the scientific revolution, and is gradually displacing folk medicine in the world; it is the dominant official medical system in every nation. Traditional medicine has developed over time, and is significantly older than modern medicine. Allopathic medicine attracts support in all ramifications (e.g., funding and research) and flourishes as a dominant healthcare system. TM, on the other hand, battles to provide basic care for large proportions of the population. The major factor explaining the displacement of TM in Africa is colonialism; European contact with Africa explains the establishment of conventional medicine as the mainstay of healthcare in Africa. Since then, coverage of conventional medicine in Africa has expanded. For many decades after independence in Africa, TM was neglected in official healthcare systems, either through a lack of formal recognition or a lack of efforts to uplift the practice.

Recently, however, there have been some important drives to foster the development and recognition of TM in Africa. The Alma-Ata Declaration, adopted by WHO and UNICEF in 1978, marked the first official recognition of the role of TM and its practitioners in primary healthcare by WHO and its Member States. Before the official declaration, there were a series of regional WHO meetings, including a meeting of African regional experts in Brazzaville in 1976, which provided some working definition of traditional medicine (see Amzat & Razum, 2014; WHO, 1976). A WHO Meeting on the Promotion and Development of Traditional Medicine was held in Geneva 1977 with a mandate of fostering ways of promoting TM (WHO, 1978). The critical themes at the Geneva meeting included integration of TM with conventional medicine in healthcare delivery; manpower development of TM; and research promotion and development in TM.

The first decade of TM in Africa was between 2001 and 2010. The second decade of TM in Africa was declared to be 2011–2020, with the hope of consolidating the achievements attained so far (WHO, 2005). The specific efforts are expected to be channeled towards policy, safety, access and rational use, with the aim of complementing the drive towards UCH in Africa. Already, it has been observed that the use of TM ranges from 70% in Benin to 90% in Burundi and Ethiopia. The advanced countries are also not left out: 42% in Belgium and 90% in the UK (WHO-Africa, 2013). While Traditional Health Practitioners (THPs) are major players in health delivery in Africa, but their specific impacts on disease control have not been adequately measured. Anyway, the THPs are significant stakeholders in disease control and management in Africa. In many African countries, herbal medicine is often used in first-line treatment of common medical conditions such fever, malaria and cough. This is because it is often readily available to prepare or purchase. The ingredients for preparing herbs are commonly sold in the market, while prepared one can also be readily bought from street vendors or hawkers.

In many communities underserved by modern health facilities (especially in rural areas), TM has been the mainstay of healthcare. The healers reside in the communities and provide affordable services to the people. It has been observed that there are more THPs in rural African communities (where over 60% resides) than modern healthcare practitioners. This implies that there is more dependence on TM especially in first-line treatment of common diseases. The contributions of TM in maternal and child health cannot be underestimated. More than 50% of deliveries in Africa take place at home. The majority of these home births are assisted by TBAs (Sialubanje, Massar, Hamer, Robert, & Ruiter, 2015). Thus training of TBAs to ensure evidence-based practice and appropriate referrals has the potential to improve delivery outcomes and maternal health in Africa.

In almost all aspects of healthcare, THPs are important caregivers providing alternative care. For instance, the scarcity of modern psychiatrists in Africa is complemented with traditional ones. Abbo (2011), in a study in Uganda, observed that traditional healers still shoulder a large burden of care of patients with mental health problems. The study concluded that since there are positive outcomes in many cases observed, it is important that traditional psychiatrists are considered in national plans for mental health. In addition, traditional medicine has helped to improve access to healthcare, especially in terms of affordability. Not only does TM contribute to healthcare, but it also contributes to the economy. In line with this, WHO-Africa (2013) observed that recorded sales of traditional medicinal products in Burkina Faso and Madagascar ranges between $3.5b and $5.3b as at year 2000. This suggests that TM is a viable economic option and can contribute to the growth of pharmaceuticals in African and around the world.

Following the realization of the relevance of traditional medicine in healthcare, there have been renewed efforts to revive it in Africa. In the year 2000, a Resolution (popularly referred to as AFR/RC50/R3, later reinforced by World Health Assembly resolution WHA62.13 in 2009) was made at the Fiftieth session of the WHO Regional Committee for Africa (Burkina Faso, 28 August–2 September 2000) (WHO, 2000). The fundamental goal was to strategize and promote TM in order to enhance its roles in the national healthcare system. WHO (2000) identified the key components of the regional strategy to include: the development of national policies, strategies and plans; capacity building; research; protection of intellectual property rights (IPRs) and traditional medicine knowledge (TMK); cultivation of medicinal plants; local production; allocation of resources; and provision of quality traditional medicine services. This document has served as a strong drive towards raising hope on the relevance of TM in the first decade of TM in Africa (2001–2010).

The series of meetings and subsequent recognition have brought back some interest in traditional medicine. Subsequent developments aimed at promoting TM in Africa and elsewhere include the *WHO Traditional Medicine Strategy 2002–2005*, the first strategy document ever prepared by WHO in this field; the traditional medicine sections of the WHO Medicines Strategy 2004–2007; and the traditional medicine components of the WHO Medicines Strategy 2008–2013. The most recent document, The *WHO Traditional Medicine Strategy 2014–2023*, harmonizes and updates the framework for action of WHO and sets the agenda for member states (WHO, 2013, p. 11). The core agenda includes:

1. Policy—integrate TM within national healthcare systems, where feasible, by developing and implementing national TM policies and programmes.
2. Safety, efficacy and quality—promote the safety, efficacy and quality of TM by expanding the knowledge base, and providing guidance on regulatory and quality assurance standards.
3. Access—increase the availability and affordability of TM, with an emphasis on access for poor populations.
4. Rational use—promote therapeutically sound use of appropriate TM by practitioners and consumers.

These four critical issues prioritized by WHO constitute the central debate in the use of TM in Africa. Having highlighted these core agenda, it is important to show an overview of responses from different African countries.

6.4   Overview of Strategies and Developments on TM in Africa

Over the past 16 years, a number of African countries have been active in uplifting the status of TM in Africa. Although slow at first, important political resolutions began in the year 2000, with the Brazzaville meeting of 1976 setting the pace for the recognition of TM by WHO. Apart from strategic documents, there was "Promoting the role of traditional medicine in health systems: A Strategy for the African Region" adopted by the WHO Regional Committee for Africa in Ouagadougou, Burkina Faso, in 2000 and the declaration on the Decade of

African Traditional Medicine (2001–2010) by the Heads of State and government in Lusaka in 2001 (WHO, 2005). The argument is always that there is need for policy formulation to regulate and promote the use of TM in Africa. Recently, serious efforts have begun to develop and implement programs to promote traditional medicine or integrate traditional and modern medicine.

Kasilo, Trapsida, Nwikisa, and Lusamba-Dikasa (2010) noted that the concept of a national policy on TM/CAM should be part of a legal framework, with objectives and strategies for achieving the set objectives. A number of African countries have already developed a legal framework for traditional medicine practice; the National Traditional Health Practitioners (THPs) Act, 2004 of South Africa; the 2010 National Codes of Ethics (NCE) for THPs, introduced in a number of countries including Ghana and Congo (Brazzaville), to enhance the safety, efficacy and quality of services provided to patients. The number with a national ethics code increased to 19 in 2012 (WHO-Africa, 2013).

Ghana is one of the leading countries in term of the regulation and promotion of TM. In 1991, the government created the Traditional Medicine Unit as part of the national Ministry of Health and has implemented a number of strategic plans to enhance the relevance and contribution of THPs (Romero-Daza, 2002). Laws and regulatory frameworks were established in 1992, and the national policy of TM was officially issued in 2002. In Ghana, there are hundreds of registered herbal medicinal products; some are sold over-the-counter. Since the enactment of regulatory frameworks, there has been laudable monitoring of herbal medicine through the Food and Drug Law Agency, which stipulates regulations regarding manufacturing, safety and marketing of herbal products in the context of medical, nutrient and health claims. A pharmacovigilance center monitors the safe use of herbal products (WHO, 2005).

In addition to Ghana, some 12 African countries have implemented national policies on TM/Complementary and Alternative Medicine (CAM), only 10 have passed laws or regulations on TM/CAM since 2005 (WHO, 2005). As of 2012, more nations have joined in the development of a national policy, increasing the number of countries to 40, while the number of countries with a legal framework increased to 28, and those with national T&CM strategic plans rose from 0 (in 1999) to 18 (WHO, 2013). Other key developments by 2010 identified by WHO (2013) include:

- There have been some developments regarding research on traditional medicine products. For instance, 28 countries were conducting research on traditional medicines for malaria, HIV/AIDS, sickle-cell anemia, diabetes and hypertension using WHO guidelines. The implication is that TM might hold some promise towards the management or cure of some well-known and widespread medical conditions.
- Thirteen countries issued marketing authorizations for traditional and complementary medicines, ranging from 3 products in Cameroon and Congo to over 1000 in Ghana and Nigeria. The media has played a key role in marketing herbal products (usually those already approved by respective Food and Drug Agencies), which have increased the demand for such products.

- Guidelines for the protection of intellectual property rights (IPR) and traditional medicine knowledge (TMK) have been developed. By 2010, nine countries had national tools for IPR and TMK protection versus zero in 1999/2000. Eight countries have established databases on traditional medicine practitioners, TMK and access to biological resources.
- Training of THPs has been intensified in many areas. For instance, there are many trained traditional birth attendants (TBAs) to deliver improved and safe services, and make appropriate referrals when necessary. Providing basic training is positive towards the integration of TM with conventional medicine.

These key developments have helped in the promotion of traditional medicine, particularly herbal medicine. Due to regulatory mechanisms, the type of traditional medicinal products that get to the public domain have been reviewed. For instance, in Nigeria, it is rare to find a media outfit advertising a herbal product without a National Agency for Food and Drug Administration and Control (NAFDAC) Number. The Number depicts official approval signifying that the product has passed through safety checks, and is therefore safe for public consumption. The Number, however, does not signify efficacy. Regulation and approval are significant in monitoring safety and adverse effects, which otherwise might be neglected. Where regulation is weak, many unverified claims float in the public domain. Research will also help to control claims from THPs. The establishment of evidence-based means that TM is moving from mere experience to experiments.

Due to some recent developments in regulation and official approval for traditional medicinal products, the progress in Ghana and Nigeria are notable. The practice of traditional medicine and the manufacturing of herbal product is turning into a booming competitive industry. Some herbal products are comparable with conventional medical products in terms of packaging and delivery. There are now herbal products in capsules and tablets or bottled with specific instructions on dosage and usage. Many registered companies are manufacturing herbal products and their derivatives for the prevention and management of various medical conditions. The inference is that the demand for herbal products, usually presented as natural products or derivatives and delivered in modern packs, might continue because of a strong local tradition towards usage of herbal products in many Africa countries. Even those that are delivered in their crude form will still continue to attract patronage because of the long traditional and cultural appeal.

6.5   Some Challenges Facing Traditional Medicine in Africa

Despite the significant progress made so far, the challenges are still enormous. There are challenges with the practice of TM itself and in the policy drive towards the recognition and promotion of the practice in healthcare delivery. The long period of neglect is responsible for some of these challenges. Perhaps if there had been considerable and consistent efforts to develop and promote TM, progress would now be further along. As it has been previously observed, the period of 2001–2010 (first decade of TM in Africa) recorded some important progress, which re-ignited the hope in TM as an alternative form of healthcare. WHO-Africa (2013) averred that some challenges hampered the implementation of the first regional traditional medicine strategy and should be better addressed in the future, especially as the continent moves to the next decade (2011–2020). Some of these critical challenges will be highlighted.

6.5.1 Problem of the "Intangible Drugs"

As previously observed, traditional medicine has both spiritual and physical aspects. While the physical aspects (mostly the resources used in herbal drugs) are amenable to science, the non-physical aspects are not. The efficacy of prayers, incantations, and appeasement of the God and gods still remain mysteries from scientific purview. Most medical remedies in biomedicine are in tangible form or in actions that are logically connected to outcomes. In TM, the diabolic or spiritual aspects are largely illogical and seem to reside in the domain of the "so-called" superior claims by the THPs. That is why in the definition of traditional medicine, the WHO also noted that TM can be "explicable or not." Understanding the non-explicable is still a major challenge, when scientific rationalism is considered.

6.5.2 Exemption of Non-Explicable Aspects of TM from Regional Efforts

Because of an emphasis on the explicable, the focus of national policies and WHO efforts is primarily herbal medicines, rather than the whole spectrum of TM. In Africa, traditional medicine goes beyond the use of herbs—in fact, herbs are a relatively small part of overall TM. Perhaps because the non-explicable is non-rational (from a biomedical point of view), most national policies and development drives significantly de-emphasized the spiritual aspects of TM. The practices of all categories of TM (traditional bone-setters, diviners, TBAs, etc.) are immersed in some constant spiritual diagnosis and remedies. This is even apart from the faith-based healers whose primary armament (against disease, infirmities and calamities) is transcendent invocation of the divine forces.

6.5.3 Weak Investment in TM

This can be explained in two ways: in budgetary allocation and research. There is little or no data on allocation to the development of TM in Africa. In general, the health sector is still poorly funded in Africa. It is not surprising that the policy and development drives in TM are not backed with adequate funding. Most of the lofty objectives in the vision 2024 for traditional medicine cannot be achieved without adequate political and economic will. There is also weak investment in terms of research. While the number of national research institutes on TM has increased to 28 (as of 2012), more direct efforts are required to uncover more herbal claims to establish Intellectual Property Right (IPR). There is a general need to mobilize THPs about the purpose and benefits of this drive and the overall objectives, bearing in mind that some THPs are non-literate. There may be thousands of herbal medicines preserved orally and through experiences that have not yet been documented. This weak investment translates to under-utilization of the potentials of THPs in Africa.

6.5.4   Poor Regulations and the Problem of Entry

The problem of entry might take a long time to solve. This is responsible for high number of charlatans with outrageous medical claims in Africa. The fake practitioners are consistently swindling the general public. It is not uncommon to find fake THPs making claims of remedies for non-curable medical conditions (such as HIV/AIDS and hypertension). While such claims cannot be simply brushed aside, the regulatory agencies should take such claims serious for credibility/efficacy checks to prevent circulation of "false" information and document breakthroughs (if any). In general, WHO-Africa (2013) noted that the uncontrolled actions of charlatans have impacted negatively on the image and credibility of traditional medicine. In many instances, there is uncontrolled street marketing of herbal products and proliferation of the use of the title "Doctor" by THPs herbal practitioners. It should, however, be noted that there have been improvements in regulatory capacities over the years, although more still needs to be done.

6.5.5   Toxicity and Safety

Beyond the registered drugs, there is proliferation of traditional medicines not registered with national food and drug agencies. Herbs are often administered for bathing, drinking and other uses. Most people continue to take the unregistered herbal products, with many ignorant of their potential toxicities (Oreagba, Oshikoya, & Amachree, 2011). It is necessary to expand efforts towards evaluating the safety, efficacy and quality of herbal medicines. There is also the need to sensitize the public on arbitrary use of herbal products whose safety and long-term effects have not been determined. Because of the paucity of research, there are no specific report about toxicity of herbal medicine, but it is high time investigations started on possible adverse effects (both in the short and long term).

6.5.6   Unethical and Unlawful Practices

Due to weak regulation, the practice of TM sometimes seems like a free-for-all practice. It is a "jungle" practice where "anything and everything" can be done. For instance, there have been reports on the use of human body parts for concoction and other spiritual remedies in many African countries (Bhootra & Weiss, 2006; Salisbury & Roberts, 2012). People living with albinism and kyphosis have been targeted for ritual and medicinal purposes responsible for the killing of over 100 albinos in Tanzania and Burundi (Cruz-Inigo, Ladizinski, & Sethi, 2011). The continuous practice of female genital mutilation is largely attributed to the THPs (although not limited to them) (Serour, 2013). The continual unethical and unlawful practices, which can also be attributed to poor regulations and weak enforcement of laws, are damaging to the image of traditional medicine. Regulating this kind of practice can help TM to take its proper place in healthcare delivery in Africa.

References

Abbo, C. (2011). Profiles and outcome of traditional healing practices for severe mental illnesses in two districts of Eastern Uganda. *Global Health Action, 4*, 7117. doi:10.3402/gha. v4i0.7117.

Abdullahi, A. A. (2011). Trends and challenges of traditional medicine in Africa. *African Journal of Traditional, Complementary, and Alternative Medicines, 8*(S), 115–123.

Amzat, J., & Razum, O. (2014). *Medical sociology in Africa.* Cham, Switzerland: Springer International Publishing.

Atwine, F., Hultsjo, S., Albin, B., Hjelm, K. (2015). Health-care seeking behaviour and the use of traditional medicine among persons with type 2 diabetes in south-western Uganda: a study of focus group interviews. *Pan African Medical Journal, 20*, 76. doi:10.11604/pamj. 2015.20.76.5497.

Bhootra, B. L., & Weiss, E. (2006). Muti killing: a case report. *Medicine, Science and the Law, 46*(3), 255–259.

Cruz-Inigo, A. E., Ladizinski, B., Sethi, A. (2011). Albinism in Africa: stigma, slaughter and awareness campaigns. *Dermatologic Clinics, 29*(1), 79–87.

Cunnama, L., & Honda, A. (2016). A mother's choice: a qualitative study of mothers' health seeking behaviour for their children with acute diarrhoea. *BMC Health Services Research, 16*, 669. doi:10.1186/s12913-016-1911-7.

Dada, A. A., Yunusa, W., Giwa, S. O. (2011). Review of the practice of traditional bone setting in Nigeria. *African Health Sciences, 11*(2), 262–265.

Elujoba, A. A., Odeleye, O. M., Ogunyemi, C. M. (2005). Traditional medicine development for medical and dental primary health care delivery system in Africa. *African Journal. Traditional, Complementary, and Alternative Medicines, 2*(1), 46–61.

Kasilo, O. M. J., Trapsida, J., Nwikisa, C. N., Lusamba-Dikasa, (2010). An overview of the traditional medicine situation in the African region. *African Health Monitor,* Issue 13.

Mahomoodally, M. F. (2013). Traditional medicines in Africa: an appraisal of ten potent African medicinal plants. *Evidence-Based Complementary and Alternative Medicine, 2013*, 617459. doi:10.1155/2013/617459.

Miles, S. H., & Ololo, H. (2003). Traditional surgeons in sub-Saharan Africa: images from south Sudan. *International Journal of STD & AIDS, 14*(8), 505–508.

Oreagba, I. A., Oshikoya, K. A., Amachree, M. (2011). Herbal medicine use among urban residents in Lagos, Nigeria. *BMC Complementary and Alternative Medicine, 11*, 117. doi:10.1186/1472-6882-11-117.

Romero-Daza, N. (2002). Traditional medicine in Africa. *Annals of the American Academy of Political and Social Science, 583*, 173–176.

Salisbury, S., & Roberts, L. (2012). The practice of ritual killings and human sacrifice in Africa. *The Human Rights Brief*, http://hrbrief.org/2012/09/the-practice-of-ritual-killings-and-human-sacrifice-in-africa/ Accessed 25 July 2016.

Serour, G. I. (2013). Medicalization of female genital mutilation/cutting. *African Journal of Urology, 19*, 145–149.

Sialubanje, C., Massar, K., Hamer, D. H., Robert, A. C., Ruiter, R. A. C. (2015). Reasons for home delivery and use of traditional birth attendants in rural Zambia: a qualitative study. *BMC Pregnancy and Childbirth, 15*, 216. doi:10.1186/s12884-015-0652-7.

Stanifer, J. W., Patel, U. D., Karia, F., Thielman, N., Maro, V., Shimbi, D., et al. (2015). The determinants of traditional medicine use in Northern Tanzania: a mixed-methods study. *PLoS One, 10*(4), e0122638. doi:10.1371/journal.pone.0122638.

WHO (1976). African traditional medicine: report of the regional expert committee. AFRO Technical Report Series, No. 1. Brazzaville.

WHO [World Health Organization] (2000). *Promoting the role of traditional medicine in health systems: a strategy for the African region*. Brazzaville: WHO.

WHO [World Health Organization] (2002). *WHO Traditional medicine strategy 2002–2005*. WHO, WHO/EDM/TRM/2002.1.

WHO [World Health Organization] (2005). *National policy on traditional medicine and regulation of herbal medicine: Report of a WHO Global Survey*. Geneva: WHO.

WHO [World Health Organization] (2013). *WHO traditional medicine strategy: 2014–2023*. Geneva: WHO.

WHO-Africa (2013). Enhancing the role of traditional medicine in health system: a strategy for the African Region. Report of Secretariat on Regional Committee Meeting, Brazzaville, Republic of Congo, 2–6 September 2013. Brazzaville: WHO.

References

114

Chapter 7
Sexual and Reproductive Health and Rights in Africa

7.1 Introduction

One of the critical areas of healthcare and rights is sexual and reproductive health and rights (SRHR). SRHR is linked to a number of health and social issues, including contraceptive use, maternal and child health, sexual transmitted diseases (STDs), family planning, population pressures, abortion, teenage pregnancy, gender equality, education, marriage and sexual and reproductive decisions, among others. It is a vital component of healthcare around the world. Investing in SRHR is key to the development agenda of any nation (Barot, 2015) and to achieving the sustainable global goals (SGDs) by 2030. IPPF (2014) also observed that SRHR cuts across the three central dimensions of sustainable development—economic, social and environmental. It is therefore important that every nation takes serious steps to ensure SRHR in order to meet development goals. While SRHR is central, it has been poorly implemented throughout the developing world. This chapter examines critical issues concerning SRHR in Africa.

7.2 What are Sexual and Reproductive Health and Rights?

SRHR is the reflection of a rights-based approach to human health and wellbeing. SRHR can be defined as the right to have control over and decide freely and responsibly on matters related to sexuality, including sexual and reproductive health, free of coercion, discrimination and violence (IPPF, 2014). The central idea is the right to self-determination in all aspects of sexuality and reproduction. SRHR is central to any development agenda.

Sexuality is "a central aspect of being human throughout life and encompasses sex, gender identities and roles, sexual orientation, eroticism, pleasure, intimacy and reproduction which is influenced by the interaction of biological, psychological,

© Springer International Publishing AG 2018

J. Amzat, O. Razum, *Towards a Sociology of Health Discourse in Africa*,
DOI 10.1007/978-3-319-61672-8_7

social, economic, political, cultural, legal, historical, religious and spiritual factors" (WHO, 2006). The cycles of sexuality include sensuality, intimacy, sexualization, sexual identity and sexual health and reproduction. Sensuality is the fulfilling pleasure; intimacy is the emotional bonding between partners; and the aspect of sexual identity contains sexual orientation including heterosexuality, homosexuality and bisexuality.

In reality, SRHR is a combination of four major concepts including sexual health, sexual rights, reproductive health and reproductive rights. In order to understand SRHR as a concept, it is important to understand each of the combining concepts.

7.2.1 What are Sexual Health and Rights?

Sexual health is "a state of physical, emotional, mental and social well-being in relation to sexuality; it is not merely the absence of disease, dysfunction or infirmity" (WHO, 2006). It requires "a positive and respectful approach to sexuality and sexual relationships, pleasurable and safe sexual experiences without coercion, discrimination and violence" (WHO, 2006). The critical aspects include avoidance of sexually transmitted diseases (STDs), unwanted pregnancy and coercive sexual experiences. It also includes sexual behaviors and sexual health seeking behavior. Sexual health is complex due to its various dimensions—physical, social, emotional and mental.

SRHR generally are within the rights context as recognized in most human right documents including the Universal Declaration of Human Rights and other international rights documents (see Box 7.1 for specific sexual rights). WHO (2006) observed that sexual rights include the right of all persons, free of coercion, discrimination and violence, to the highest attainable standard of sexual health. Generally, it is the application of human rights to sexuality, or sexual health in particular. Like the right to health, there must be commitment to respect, protect and fulfill sexual rights.

Box 7.1 Specific sexual rights
- Access to sexual and reproductive health care services;
- Seek, receive and impart information related to sexuality;
- Access to sexuality education;
- Respect for bodily integrity;
- Choose their partner;
- Decide to be sexually active or not;
- Have consensual sexual relations;
- Consensual marriage;
- Decide whether or not, and when, to have children; and
- Pursue a satisfying, safe and pleasurable sexual life.

Source WHO (2006)

7.2.2   Reproductive Health and Rights

The concept of reproductive health and rights (RHR) is closely related to sexual health—they are obviously interwoven. Why it is sometimes separated from sexual health is that reproduction involves more issues. Reproductive health is a state of complete physical, mental and social well-being, and not merely the absence of reproductive disease or infirmity. Reproductive health addresses the reproductive processes, functions and system at all stages of life. According to WHO, reproductive health, therefore, implies that people are able to have a responsible, satisfying and safe sex life and that they have the capability to reproduce and the freedom to decide if, when and how often to do so. This includes desire to have children or not, the number, timing and spacing of children, informed decision to access contraceptive/ family planning services, and maternal and child care, assisted births, prevention of STI, safe and post-abortion care and information relating to reproduction.

Reproductive rights are recognized in international human rights documents. It only applies to reproduction to signify freedom from all forms of issues inimical to reproductive rights. The right to determine freely all aspects of relating to number, timing and spacing of children and access to reproductive activities including appropriate reproductive services to attaining the highest standard of reproductive health. The 1994 International Conference on Population and Development in Cairo (ICPD) has been the major reference in the declaration of reproductive rights. The ICPD (1994) further declared that in the exercise of this right, individuals should take into account the needs of their living and future children and their responsibilities towards the community (UNFPA, 2004). This simply implies responsible parenthood. This is the reason behind planned parenthood, that people should take control and act within their limit or carrying capacity regarding family size or fertility preference.

7.3   The State of Sexual and Reproductive Health and Rights in Africa

In addition to the Universal Declaration of Human Rights (Article 25) in 1948, The International Covenant on Economic, Social and Cultural Rights (Article 12) in 1976, and The African Charter on Human and Peoples' Rights (Article 16) in 1981, which all include the right to health, the 1994 ICPD signifies a major landmark in the entrenchment of SRHR all over the world. The ICPD is an attempt to further explicate SRHR from the general framework already existing in various conventions, and even the conception of health in general. The (African) Continental Policy Framework on Sexual and Reproductive Health and Rights was developed in Botswana in 2005 (following a series of regional meetings between 2004 and 2005) and endorsed by the Summit of the African Heads of State and Government in Khartoum, Sudan in 2006 (AUC, 2006).

The previous MDGs and the new global goals also include targets relating to SRHR. There is also the "Addis Ababa Declaration on Population and Development in Africa beyond 2014" which reaffirmed the commitment towards ensuring SRHR in Africa. As previously mentioned, SRHR relates to a number of fundamental issues, some of which will be briefly examined. For the purpose of this section, same-sex relationships, contraception, and maternal health issues will be discussed.

7.3.1 Same-Sex Relationships/Unions in Africa

One aspect of SRHR is the freedom to choose a partner of any sex or gender. Legal protections for people in same-sex relationships are far from established, either globally, or in Africa. As of the end of 2016, only South Africa and Seychelles have some legal provision protecting same-sex relationship among adults. Most African countries continue to criminalize these relationships, with punishments ranging from life sentence in Uganda, Tanzania and Sierra Leone, to death sentences in Somalia, Sudan and Libya. In many other States (including Liberia, Algeria, Egypt, Botswana, Malawi, Mauritius, Senegal, Zambia, Eritrea, Tunisia, Togo, Morocco and Ethiopia), the punishment can range from 1 to 20 years imprisonment. Even in those countries (including Cape Verde, Benin, Madagascar, Niger, Rwanda, Cote d'Ivoire and Djibouti) where same-sex relationships are not criminalized, they are still not legally recognized (see The Library of Congress, 2014). In most States where same-sex relationship is criminalized, it is regarded as sodomy, indecent act or unnatural offence.

In the arena of international conventions, criminalization of same-sex unions signifies an infraction of sexual rights. Although gradual advocacy for the rights of sexual minorities in Africa is gaining traction, including some open demonstration against discriminatory laws in most instances, same-sex couples are stigmatized and may even face "jungle justice" (like mob action, i.e., people acting violently against same-sex partners or their property) when they display affection in public. In nearly all African countries, homosexual communities exist as minority group without a voice.

Discriminatory laws against same-sex couples are extremely restrictive. In Nigeria, for example, a bill prohibiting same-sex marriage that was signed into law in 2014, also placed embargoes on their freedom of assembly, speech, and association. The law further prohibits any advocacy and open gathering in the name of sexual rights for the affected group. Such laws can have health implications: Lesbian, gay, bisexual, and transgender groups (LGBT) communities often undergo minority stress with attendant psychosocial implications (see McAdams-Mahmoud et al., 2014). In addition, there is significantly compromised healthcare delivery and adverse health outcomes among LGBT community (Buffie, 2011). Same-sex couples are completely excluded from the benefits of legal marital unions. Beyrer (2014) observed that LGBT communities bear disproportionate burdens of HIV risk and face stigma and discrimination in accessing needed health services (see also Barnett-Vanes, 2014). It is further observed that the current wave of anti-gay laws and policies are likely to reduce access to healthcare, increase discrimination, and impact HIV research and programs. Antigay policies and laws are infractions of the SRHR and, by implication, against the right to health and other fundamental human rights.

7.3.2   Contraception: The Unmet Need

Contraception, also known as birth control or fertility control, is a means of preventing or delaying pregnancy as a consequence of sexual intercourse. Africa is a continent with high fertility and low contraceptive use. This has a good deal to do with socio-economic development. Globally, use of modern contraception has risen from 54% in 1990 to 57.4% in 2014. In Africa, the proportion of women aged 15–49 using contraceptives rose from 23.6% to 27.6%, in Asia it has risen slightly from 60.9% to 61.6%, and in Latin America and the Caribbean, it rose slightly from 66.7% to 67.0% (WHO, 2016). Contraception should be universally available, since it is needed by most of the adult population. The problem is that there is still unmet need in contraceptive use.

Access to contraception is a major component of sexual health and rights. It aids individuals in self-determining whether to become pregnant and the timing of pregnancies, including the spacing of children. Poor maternal health is closely related to pregnancy that comes too early or too often. With the use of contraception, pregnancy can be delayed or stopped without interfering in normal sexual relations. The use of contraceptives reduces pregnancy-related morbidity and mortality and related to better birth outcomes. Generally, the population figure is often compared with carrying capacity of the society, i.e., at household level, the family socio-economic resources should be able to support the number of household members. Contraption helps to limit the number of children to a number the couple can adequately support. This helps to limit family size to a number that can be adequately supported.

Across African countries, there is high unmet need for contraception. Unmet need signifies the number of those who require contraception but lack information on or access to it. Unmet needs also points to the gap between women's reproductive intentions and their contraceptive behavior. This is why in many parts of the world unwanted/unplanned pregnancy remains very high. For instance, it was reported that worldwide in 2012, 85 million pregnancies, representing 40% of all pregnancies, were unintended. Of these, 50% ended in abortion, 13% ended in miscarriage, and 38% resulted in an unplanned birth (Sedgh, Singh, & Hussain, 2014). Unintended pregnancies can have economic and psychosocial implications. Due to unintended pregnancies, many young girls have to spend many years out of school to care for pregnancy, and later the baby. Many of them might not be able to return to school. This is apart from the difficulties experienced in sourcing for livelihood for the baby. Some of those girls are teenagers, who do not have any means of livelihood. The growth of the foetus in most instances is hampered right from pregnancy and afterwards because of inadequate maternal feeding.

Beyond the economic impact, unmet need for contraception can have fatal consequences. For instance, many women who have unplanned pregnancy resorts to abortion, resulting in a number of death partly because of restrictive abortion laws in Africa. In general, there are restrictive abortion laws in most African countries, even in a few countries where abortion is permitted under certain circumstance; access to such service is difficult (Guttmacher, 2016). Out of 54 African countries, only five (Zambia, Cape Verde, Mozambique, South Africa and Tunisia) have relatively liberal abortion laws. In Angola, Central African Republic, Congo (Brazzaville), Democratic Republic of the Congo, Egypt, Gabon, Guinea-Bissau, Madagascar, Mauritania, São Tomé and Principe, Senegal and Somalia, abortion is strictly prohibited, with no explicit legal exception to save the life of a woman (Guttmacher, 2016).

Restrictions on abortions lead to illegal and unsafe abortions. Almost all abortion-related deaths worldwide occur in developing countries, with the highest number occurring in Africa. Globally, unsafe abortions are responsible for at least 9% of maternal deaths (16,000) annually (Guttmacher, 2016). In Africa, between 2010 and 2014, an estimated 8.3 million induced abortions occurred each year. Variation by region ranged from 38 per 1,000 women of childbearing age in North Africa to 31 per 1,000 in West Africa, and 34 per 1,000 in East, Middle and southern Africa (Guttmacher, 2016; Sedgh et al., 2016).

Unfortunately, many of these countries with strict abortion laws do not consider it as violation of SRHR. This is because such laws are sanctioned with some cultural and religious norms. Apparently, such restrictive abortion laws hold adverse implications for SRHR.

7.3.3 Maternal Health

The state of maternal health is still very poor in Africa, and the rate of maternal mortality remains high. The maternal mortality ratio (MMR [maternal deaths per 100,000 live births]) is still 546 and 70 for SSA and North Africa respectively (WHO, 2015). Most countries with high estimated MMR are in Africa (see Box 7.2). It is further observed that Nigeria (a country with the highest population in Africa) accounts for the highest number of deaths in 2015 with an approximate 58,000 maternal deaths constituting 19% (see Box 7.2 for MMR in some other African countries). The general data from SSA is an increase from previous estimates of 510 in 2013 (WHO, 2014). Nigeria's estimate was also 560 as at 2013. This could imply that the situation is getting worst instead of improving. The central concern is that this high MMR is connected to human rights issues.

Box 7.2 Maternal Mortality Ratio in African States

Sierra Leone	1360
Central African Republic	882
Chad	856
Nigeria	814
South Sudan	789
Somalia	732
Liberia	725
Burundi	712
Gambia	706
D. R. Congo	693
Guinea	679
Côte d'Ivoire	645
Malawi	634
Mauritania	602
Cameroon	596
Mali	587
Niger	553
Guinea- Bissau	549
Kenya	510
Mauritius	53
Cape Verde	42

Source WHO (2016)

Maternal health is a further building block of SRHR. Maternal health refers to women's health during pregnancy, childbirth and the postpartum period. WHO noted that while motherhood should be a positive event, it is sometimes associated with suffering and death. With reference of right to health, maternal health is often stressed as a human right. There have been some landmark events, such as Convention on the Elimination of All Forms of Discrimination against Women (CEDAW) in 1979; the 1994 ICPD (Cairo); and the 1995 Fourth World Conference on Women (Beijing) regarding women's health and human rights (see Gruskin et al., 2008; Yamin, 2013). Those efforts represent movements to activate the connection between human rights discourse and maternal health, morbidity and mortality. Despite human right movements, certain cultural realities continue to exhibit social contradictions that are unfavorable to women in terms of reproductive rights (and maternal health) because most of those treaties and international laws are weakly implemented or not domesticated at all (Amzat, 2015).

The crux is that rights concerns are associated with negative outcomes in maternal health in Africa (Amzat, 2015). The first concern is that the rights of women to have control over their bodies. Such control is often compromised by certain sociocultural norms hence such right is not adequately protected by law. Other major issues relate to limited access to paid employment and relative care. All these often compromise maternal health. This is why morbidity and mortality is relatively high in Africa. It has been observed that the high rate of maternal mortality in Africa is a reflection of human right violations entrenched through certain cultural and legal norms, which promote discrimination and relative care. Such harmful social norms and practices affect women throughout lifetime including child marriage, forced marriage, wife battery, household inequality, deprivation of education and inheritance, limited access to paid employment, feminisation of poverty among others.

Applying the rights-based approach by protecting women's rights against all forms of discriminatory and unjust norms, will help tremendously to revert the scandalous MMR across African countries (especially SSA) and elsewhere. Impliedly, the rights-based approach will help to address "the underlying power relations that systematically put women—some more than others—at risk of SRHR violations, and MMM [maternal morbidity and mortality] in particular, and enabling women to live lives of dignity" (Yamin, 2013, p. 1). This is possibly addressed within the health system, and more importantly, beyond the system as many of the issues are community matters.

7.4   Social Determinants of SRHR in Africa

Having discussed some critical health issues relating to SRHR, it is important to further explore some specific and fundamental sociocultural contexts—or simply put—social determinants of SRHR in Africa. There are a number of underlying social issues shaping SRHR in Africa, most of which are cultural, political and organizational. They are the vectors to be addressed if SRHR is to be fulfilled and protected. Some of those determinants (including culture, education, economic factor, health system, legal and policy context, sexual violence and coercion) will be examined.

7.4.1   The Sociocultural Context of SRHR

The sociocultural context is like a wellspring from which flow a number of factors that fundamentally shape SRHR in Africa and elsewhere. Impliedly, the context is a complex whole including religion, gender, patriarchy, marriage pattern, traditional practices and whole lot of other issues. The context generates norms penetrating every sector of the society, from the family unit to the public realm. Those norms invariably affect SRHR in the society. The sociocultural context dictates the gender norm in the society. Where inequality or unbalance power relation between the sexes is sanctioned, like in the African context, women bear the brunt of the inequality. In most cases, woman body is a contested entity; she is often deprived of its ownership. In most African societies, the female body within marriage is perceived to be "owned" by her husband. Hence, the male partner exercises control over the body—defining, in most instances, all matters relating to SRHR. Decisions regarding family size, availability for sex, use of contraceptives, and even health-seeking behavior are usually within the domain of men. Such situation is inimical to SRHR, as the body bearer is the owner and should decide on all matters affecting the body.

Most of these gender norms are sanctioned by religion. For instance, Islam and Christianity preach submissiveness of the wife to the husband, and that a man should be the breadwinner. Invariably, most gender norms are also rationalized as religious dictates, and Africa is a religious continent. Islam and most African cultures allow multiple marital partnerships called polygyny when a man marries more than one wife simultaneously. A study found that polygyny is associated with an accelerated transmission of STIs because of multiplication of sexual partners, low rates of condom use, poor communication between spouses, among other factors (Bove & Valeggia, 2009). Polygyny is also associated with premature "social" menopause (a kind of self-withdrawal from major social activities including sexual activities) (Bove & Valeggia, 2009). It makes marriage a kind of competition among co-wives, which could invariably affect their general well-being including mental state. For most Pentecostals in Africa, marriage is an enduring union without option of divorce (for the couple). A woman or man has to endure all the pains (most times including assaults).

Some cultural practices also hold implication for SRHR in Africa. The practices of forced and child marriage are also pervasive. This marriage pattern is non-consensual and puts child-wives at a dehumanizing state within the marital union. A child is still growing, with physiology not prepared for the demands (including sex, house chores, etc.) of marriage, and then has to be denied childhood and forced into marriage usually with a man much older. This is apparent denial of SRHR. In many cultures, puberty (or even onset of menstruation) is perceived as maturity, which could mean marriage and end of schooling for girls (WHO, 2006, 2010). Puberty also comes with a number of traditional rites including forced fattening and female genital cutting in many cultures.

Some cultures also exact undue pressure on men as the breadwinners of the family. Under such circumstances, maleness means toughness and ability to exact control on women. Many cultures promote this dominance motivation, which encourages aggression or violence against women. A common male ideology is that which permits multiple sexual partnerships for men, which increases male vulnerability to STIs. The implication is that there are a lot of cultural values and norms, which limit individual's ability to have safe, equitable and consensual sexual and reproductive relations. Such norms and values constitute infringement on the rights of individuals (both male and female). Although in most circumstances, especially due to patriarchy, women bear the brunt of unjust sociocultural norms in African societies. Sociocultural context, therefore, holds significant implications for SRHR.

7.4.2 Economic Milieu of SRHR

Economic status is a major determinant of health in general, and in particular, significantly affects SRHR. This section will mainly focus on poverty, a state of economic deprivation or inadequate basic needs for survival. Poverty rate is still very high in Africa. It has been observed that poverty is correlated with poor reproductive health indicators including maternal survival, early child bearing, unintended pregnancy, unsafe abortion, shorter birth interval, and child mortality (Rao, Gopalakrishnan, Kuruvilla, & Jacob, 2012). It limits access to maternal health services. Other poor sexual and reproductive health indicators are common among the poor. This is because poverty makes people vulnerable to all sorts of sexual health concerns. For instance, poverty is a major factor pushing some African women into commercial sex work, which is illegal in most African countries. Women are also victims of sexual assaults (including rape) when in search of means of livelihood.

Poverty and SRHR has a bidirectional relationship; poverty contributes to poor SRHR, and poor SRHR also contributes to poverty. For most women, poverty is strongly correlated with early pregnancy and child bearing (Green & Merrick, 2005), which are also correlated with poor educational attainment and low labor participation, and hence, poor socio-economic condition. Sinding (2005) noted that where reproductive rights are realized, fertility and population growth decline, and individual and societal prosperity are enhanced. Where people are able to take informed decision about their sexual and reproductive activities, they are likely to make healthy choices. Fertility rate often declines with rising prosperity or development. This partly explains why population growth rate is high in developing world and low in developed world.

Poverty is one of the structures, which regulates people's sexual practices and constraints (Jolly, 2010). Commercialization of sex is widespread (most times associated with poverty), often with little or no power to negotiate safe sex. The poor are likely to give out an underage female in marriage in return for financial gains or freedom from financial responsibility. Poverty can also make people more vulnerable to abuses of sexual rights (Jolly, 2010). For instance, a report by Baobab for Women's Human Rights indicated that most of those charged under sharia laws in northern Nigeria were poor, usually rural, or urban poor and non-literates—mostly charged for adultery or fornication (Jolly, 2010). The preceding example also represents unequal application of laws

Economic status also affects how people negotiate sexuality norms. Efforts towards reducing poverty will enhance SRHR and vice-versa. This will impact on many SRHR issues including early marriage, sexual violence, maternal health-seeking behavior, sexual lifestyles, and women empowerment. Addressing all these through enhancement of SRHR will also impact on overall national development.

7.4.3   Education and Health Literacy as Determinants of SRHR

Education involves general acquisition of skills, knowledge and values, which can be applied in daily life. It is so connected with health literacy, which also involves the ability to obtain, understand and use basic health information in manners that will enhance better health outcomes. Education is a foundation of health literacy. Education and health literacy help to strengthen agency (Razum, Weishaar, & Schaeffer, 2016), ensuring that individual make informed decision that would lead to better health outcomes. It begins with awareness of basic information about hygiene, preventive measures, disease condition, appropriate care seeking patterns and other health-related issues. Education is a basic foundation of SRHR because it helps individuals to acquire basic knowledge of SRHR. A right is better claimed when individuals are aware of it. This is why it is fundamentally important for everyone to have some knowledge of SRHR right from childhood—appropriated to age as much as possible.

It has been argued that reaching people with SRHR education right from school is a good starting point. SRHR education among young persons will help to reduce "misinformation and increase accurate knowledge; clarify and strengthen positive values and attitudes; increase the skills needed to make informed decisions and act upon them; improve perceptions about peer groups and social norms; and increase communication with parents or other trusted adults" (Wahab & Roudi-Fahimi, 2012, p. 3). For instance, Tunisia was acknowledged as the first Muslim country to introduce information on reproduction and family planning in its school curriculum since the early 1960s, and in the 1990s, it introduced reproductive health education for both girls and boys also in public school curriculum (Wahab & Roudi-Fahimi, 2012).

Education is important because its low level is correlated with poor SRHR outcomes (Erinosho, 2014). Education often impacts positively on several measures of SRHR: sexual initiation, contraceptive use, likelihood of pregnancy, probability of contracting a sexually transmitted disease, early marriage and child bearing, number of children, negotiation of safer sex, maternal health outcomes, and child health (see Doyle, Mavedzenge, Plummer, & Ross, 2012; Esere, 2008). Education improves self-efficacy to negotiate and implement safer sexual relationships among other benefits. Education is therefore a major determinant of health. Improving literacy rate means empowering the people to access information and skills that will be vital to survival. This will impact positively on health indicators in general and SRHR in particular.

7.4.4   Roles of the Health Systems

One major factor shaping health in general is the health systems; the way health systems are designed, operated and financed act as a powerful determinant of health (Gilson, Doherty, Loewenson, & Francis, 2007). The primary role of the health systems is to improve health. Health system is about workforce, health financing, health information, service delivery and medicines (see Sect. 1.5)—all put together affect population health. The broad range of services provided regarding SRHR might determine the SRHR of the population. It requires the health system to provide comprehensive services to the population in manners accessible to all. Non-availability of some services (regarding SRHR) signifies a disservice to the community and might indicate some negative effects. It also requires that the health systems provide appropriate information to the community. This is a definite way of influencing the health literacy level of the population.

When it comes to SRHR, the professionalism and attitude of the providers are very important. Issues of sexuality are often sensitive; it requires some rigorous ethical considerations, without which services might not be accessed. Rao et al. (2012) observed that confidential and nondiscriminatory health services with preventive, curative, counseling and referral services should be available to all. Privacy is a major ethical issue in SRHR; where privacy is lax, services might be underutilized. Providers' attitude can encourage or discourage use of sexual and reproductive health services. The technical competence of staff including cultural competence and interpersonal relations are very important in SRHR services. In most instances, women most often prefer to be examined by a female provider when care involves vagina examination. In African countries, where preserving women's modesty is paramount, fear of having one's body exposed to others (especially opposite sex) can prevent women from obtaining SRHR services (WHO, 2010).

In general, the health systems determine SRHR of a community. Services should be tailored to the needs of the community. Services should also be client-centered. Cultural norms that promote respect and dignity of the client should be technically observed in order to promote service utilization. And more importantly, norms promoting inequity must be competently addressed. Adequate fund and effective medicines and technologies must be made available to facilitate effective care delivery. These are sure ways the health system affect general healthcare delivery, and SRHR in particular.

7.4.5   Legal and Policy Context of SRHR

Beyond general human rights entrenched in national constitutions, there are also policies and specific laws relating to SRHR. This greatly determines SRHR in every state. For instance, legal and policy framework includes specific laws and policies such as population/fertility policy, abortion laws, sexual offences Acts, marriage and family laws among others, which affect SRHR. Most countries now have laws on same-sex union (see Sect. 7.3.1) and abortion (see Sect. 7.3.2)—there is outright denial of those "rights" in many African countries. Many countries have stipulated punishment for any infraction on sexual health and rights. The policy and legal environment often dictate the possibilities, prohibitions and goals regarding SRHR. Specifically, the policy environment affects barriers to services for SRHR, access to essential medicines, healthcare providers' obligation, criminalization of sexual-health-related services, implementation of ethical principles (privacy, confidentiality and informed consent) among others.

The central concerns regarding the policy and legal environment is whether (1) national laws/policies give recognition to SRHR; (2) some specific issues are addressed through law/policies; (3) implementation strategies are spelt out and followed; and (4) goals are specifically set. It is however important to understand the direction of those laws and policies—whether they are supportive of SRHR or not, and their overall impacts over a period of time. Laws against sexual violence such as rape (including marital rape) hate/honor crimes; and sexual exploitation (including trafficking of minors/women) have been very supportive in promoting SRHR. Laws against sexual assaults, discrimination/stigma and gender inequality-gender inequality are also promotive of SRHR.

The policy environment should address access to SRHR services, including availability, affordability, acceptability and quality of sexual health services (e.g., services for abortion, contraception, STI prevention, testing and treatment). The policy environment should also address vulnerable groups such as commercial sex workers, youths, military, and trafficked persons. For instance, Kenya (like many other African countries) has National Adolescent Reproductive Health Policy meant to enhance equitable access to high quality, efficient and effective adolescent friendly sexual and reproductive information and services among others objective. Population control is also a major target of every nation. In most African countries, the target is to reduce population growth rate. By implication, the policy and legal measures are imperative for full realization of SRHR.

7.4.6 Sexual Violence and Coercion

Sexual violence (SV) is singled out as a major determinant of SRHR. Sexual violence (such as including rape, sexual abuse of children and forced marriage and other sexual exploitation) is highly prevalent around the world. Sexual violence heightens the risk of STIs, and in general, it is a dehumanizing experience. This is why WHO considered sexual violence as a serious public health and human rights problem with both short- and long-term consequences on physical, mental, and sexual and reproductive health of every individual (although women are the most affected). SV refers to sexual activity when consent is not obtained or freely obtained. One of the pressing concerns is that some violent acts (wife battery, child marriage and marital rape) are culturally tolerated in many instances (see Alesina, Brioschi, & Ferrara, 2016). Such social toleration is partially responsible for the poor SRHR indicators.

While the legal framework can play protective role, influencing cultural norms is a major challenge in Africa. Some of those cultural norms are sustained over the years, though some changes are being observed. There is still the need to address culturally sanctioned gender-based violence which impact on SRHR. Even where there is no cultural tolerance, violent acts are still prevalent. In general, there must be protective mechanisms for the entire population in general and the vulnerable population in particular.

References

African Union Commission (AUC) (2006). *Sexual and reproductive health and rights: continental policy framework*. AU: Addis Ababa.

Alesina, A., Brioschi, B., Ferrara, E. (2016). Violence against women: a cross-cultural analysis for Africa. Cambridge: National Bureau of Economic Research, NBER Working Paper, 21901.

Amzat, J. (2015). The question of autonomy in maternal health: a rights-based consideration. *Journal of Bioethical Inquiry, 15*(2), 283–293. doi:10.1007/s11673-015-9607-y.

Barnett-Vanes, A. (2014). Criminalising homosexuality threatens the fight against HIV/AIDS. *Lancet, 383*, 783–784.

Barot, S. (2015). Sexual and reproductive health and rights are key to global development: the case for ramping up investment. *Guttmacher Policy Review, 18*(1), 1–7.

Beyrer, C. (2014). Pushback: the current wave of anti-homosexuality laws and impacts on health. *PLoS Medicine, 11*(6), e1001658. doi:10.1371/journal.pmed.1001658.

Bove, R., & Valeggia, C. (2009). Polygyny and women's health in sub-Saharan Africa. *Social Science & Medicine, 68*(1), 21–29.

Buffie, W. C. (2011). Public health implications of same-sex marriage. *American Journal of Public Health, 101*(6), 986–990. doi:10.2105/AJPH.2010.300112.

Doyle, A. M., Mavedzenge, S. N., Plummer, M. L., Ross, D. A. (2012). The sexual behaviour of adolescents in sub-Saharan Africa: patterns and trends from national surveys. *Tropical Medicine & International Health, 17*(7), 796–807.

Erinosho, O. (2014). Social determinant of sexual reproductive health in Africa. In F. Okonofua (Ed.) *Confronting the challenge of reproductive health in Africa: a textbook for students and development practitioners*. Florida: BrownWalker Press.

Esere, M. O. (2008). Effect of sex education programme on at-risk sexual behaviour of school-going adolescents in Ilorin, Nigeria. *African Health Sciences, 8*(2), 120–125.

Gilson, L., Doherty, J., Loewenson, R., Francis, V. (2007). Challenging inequity through the health systems. Final Report Knowledge Network on Health Systems June 2007. WHO, Geneva: Commission on Social Determinants of Health.

Green, M. E. & Merrick, T. (2005). Poverty reduction: does reproductive health matter? Washington, DC: The International Bank for Reconstruction and Development/The World Bank (Health, Nutrition and Population (HNP) Discussion Paper).

Gruskin, S., Cottingham, J., Hilber, A. M., Kismodi, E., Lincetto, O., Roseman, M. J. (2008). Using human rights to improve maternal and neonatal health: history, connections and a proposed practical approach. *Bulletin of the World Health Organization, 86*(8), 589–593. doi:10.2471/BLT.07.050500.

Guttmacher (2016). *Fact Sheet: abortion in Africa*. New York: Guttmacher.

IPPF (2014). *Sexual and reproductive health and rights—a crucial agenda for the post-2015 framework*. London: IPPF.

Jolly, S. (2010). Poverty and sexuality: what are the connections? An overview of the literatures. Stockholm: Swedish International Development Cooperation Agency.

McAdams-Mahmoud, A., Stephenson, R., Rentsch, C., Cooper, H., Arriola, K. J., Jobson, G., et al. (2014). Minority stress in the lives of men who have sex with men in Cape Town, South Africa. *Journal of Sexuality, 61*(6), 847–867.

Rao, T. S., Gopalakrishnan, R., Kuruvilla, A., Jacob, K. S. (2012). Social determinants of sexual health. *Indian Journal of Psychiatry, 54*(2), 105–107.

Razum, O., Weishaar, H., Schaeffer, D. (2016). Health literacy: strengthening agency or changing structures? *International Journal of Public Health, 61*, 277–278.

Sedgh, G., Bearak, J., Singh, S., Bankole, A., Popinchalk, A., Ganatra, B., et al. (2016). Abortion incidence between 1990 and 2014: global, regional, and subregional levels and trends. *Lancet, 388*, 258–267. doi:10.1016/S0140-6736(16)30380-4.

Sedgh, G., Singh, S., Hussain, R. (2014). Intended and unintended pregnancies worldwide in 2012 and recent trends. *Studies in Family Planning, 45*(3), 301–314.

Sinding, S. W. (2005). Keeping sexual and reproductive health at the forefront of global efforts to reduce poverty. *Studies in Family Planning, 36*(2), 140–143.

The Library of Congress (2014). Laws on homosexuality in African Nations. https://www. loc.gov/law/help/criminal-laws-on-homosexuality/homosexuality-laws-in-african-nations.pdf. Accessed 24 May 2016.

UNPFA (2004). Program of action adopted at the international conference on population and development, 5–13 September 1994. New York: United Nations Population Fund.

Wahab, M., & Roudi-Fahimi, F. (2012). The need for reproductive health education in schools in Egypt. Washington, D.C: Policy Brief, Population Reference Bureau.

World Health Organisation (WHO) (2006). Defining sexual health: report of a technical consultation on sexual health, 28–31 January 2002. Geneva, World Health Organization.

World Health Organisation (WHO) (2010). *Social determinants of sexual and reproductive health: informing future research and programme implementation / edited by Shawn Malarcher.* Geneva: WHO.

World Health Organization (WHO) (2014). *Trends in maternal mortality: 1990 to 2013: estimates by WHO, UNICEF, UNFPA, The World Bank and the United Nations Population Division.* Geneva: WHO.

World Health Organisation (WHO) (2015). *Trends in maternal mortality: 1990 to 2013: estimates by WHO, UNICEF, UNFPA, The World Bank and the United Nations Population Division.* Geneva: WHO.

World Health Organisation (WHO) (2016). Family planning/Contraception Fact sheet. No 351 http://who.int/mediacentre/factsheets/fs351/en/. Accessed 24 May 2016.

Yamin, A. E. (2013). From ideals to tools: applying human rights to maternal health. *PLoS Medicine, 10*(11), e1001546. doi:10.1371/journal.pmed.1001546.

Chapter 8
Rural Health in Africa

8.1 Introduction

Rural health is emerging as a distinct field of study with a multi-disciplinary approach (including the fields medicine, sociology, nursing, geography, etc.), focusing on health and healthcare delivery in rural areas. The main discourse in the field is to examine the multifactorial complexities accounting for the state of global rural health. From the most advanced country to the poorest one, intra-country rural-urban health disparities are evident. The essence of this chapter is to focus on rural health conditions (especially in Africa), which incidentally constitutes one of the priorities of rural medicine. Rural health is part of the larger discourse on healthcare in Africa. This is because the African region has up to 60% of its population residing in rural areas and up to 80% of the rural population face some extreme difficulties in accessing modern healthcare, despite pressing needs.

One of the fundamental challenges in healthcare in Africa is how to cover the rural areas. Africa is still largely rural (up to 60%). In terms of healthcare, those in the rural areas are grossly underserved with health services. Coverage of both urban and rural areas is still a major challenge, but the relative and greater brunt of poor healthcare coverage is borne by the rural areas where more than 60% of the people reside. This is a geographical dimension of health inequalities that have persisted over the years. It highlights the importance of place (of residence) as a determinant of health. Spatial location is a major factor in health. In this regard, location or space, whether rural or urban, exact significance influence on population health. Because Africa is largely rural, it is significant to examine the healthcare of the rural dwellers. If wider coverage is a target, then the health of the rural dwellers should be a major focus. While this would require huge resources, it is a worthwhile adventure in order to ensure UHC and to fulfill health as human right.

Rural healthcare in Africa is severely inadequate. The international labor organization (ILO) worked on the global disparities between the rural and urban, and provided first time global evidence that shows "significant if not extreme

© Springer International Publishing AG 2018
J. Amzat, O. Razum, *Towards a Sociology of Health Discourse in Africa*,
DOI 10.1007/978-3-319-61672-8_8

differences between rural and urban populations in health coverage" (Scheil-Adlung/ILO, 2015). It is extreme to the extent that in many rural communities of Africa, modern health facilities are non-existent. This is largely due to urban bias in the distribution of health facilities in many nations. Both private and public health institutions are often sited in urban areas at the neglect of the rural areas. Scheil-Adlung/ILO (2015) observed that while 56% of the global rural population lacks health coverage, only 22% of the urban population is not covered. While this is a global picture, the situation is often worse in Africa.

Rural healthcare is a major health discourse in Africa because almost 70% of morbidities and mortalities from major disease burden occur in rural Africa. This has been the trend over the years; rural health has often been met with lip service. The trend is alarming because of the poor healthcare situation and worsening determinants of health. The rural African communities often show a place of gross deprivations, which are detrimental to population health. This deprivation complex (of healthcare facilities and other related factors) accounts for poor health status in rural areas of Africa. For instance, Scheil-Adlung/ILO (2015) observed that rural maternal mortality is 2.5 times higher than urban rates. The inequality in suffering and death is a socio-political creation due to long time neglect of the rural areas. This is why rural health is a major health discourse in Africa. Therefore, this chapter will examine some critical issues connected to rural health in Africa. The chapter will also examine the state of healthcare in rural Africa, the characters of rural communities and the basis of healthcare challenge in rural African communities.

8.2   Features of Rural Communities

African rural communities are typically underdeveloped settlements. Underdevelopment in this sense is a relative term, focusing on the relative notion of modern or developed communities. Defining a rural community is often relative and also bothers on a number of criteria including population density, number of households or population size, social amenities, and sometimes, socio-political judgments. A definition can include a number of these criteria, or there could be a political or policy dimension in defining a rural settlement. A simple definition stipulates that any place that is not considered an urban area is adjudged as a rural area. This will lead to double task of defining an urban area, then differentiating it from a rural one. But this, perhaps, helps to make a simple clarification: any place that is outside of the city or town is rural. The rural is sometimes called the countryside or remote area.

"A rural area is a sparsely populated area in which people farm or depend on natural resources, including hamlets, villages and small towns" (Dala-Clayton, Dent, & Dubois, 2013). Therefore, a rural area is a place with low population density and that is outside the urban region. In Africa, rural areas are scattered settlements across vast land mostly remotely located and underserved with basic social amenities. In a critical turn, Tekeuchi (2016) defined "rural" in the notion of "rural development" as a place where the poor live. This could be right to the extent that rural life has a face of poverty (at least in Africa) as up to 70% of the poor live there. Because there are still urban poor, poverty cannot really be the only yardstick in defining rural life. In reality, cities grow out of rural areas, and urbanization has been a major drive in the modern world. While rural population size might continue to diminish due to rural-urban migration, it will take several decades in Africa before there would be an even population distribution. Table 8.1 shows the rural-urban population in Africa with a projection up to 2025.

The Table further shows that Africa is largely rural with almost 60% of its population living in rural areas. While the continent is urbanizing, the rural population is expected to be higher for several more years. It is, however, projected to be slightly less than urban dwellers by 2050 (UN, 2015). As shown in Table 8.1, Southern African and Northern Africa are the most urbanized in Africa, with 61.6% and 51.6%, respectively. In the other regions, rural dwellers are substantially higher than urban dwellers. East Africa is the most rural of all regions, with 74.4% of its population residing in rural areas. In general, it has been observed that the process of urbanization is associated with important economic and social transformations, which have brought greater geographic mobility, lower fertility, longer life expectancy and population ageing (UN, 2015). The urban center has been a symbol of development and poverty reduction as it attracts substantial national economic and political activities supported with high level of infrastructure. The opposite seems to be the case for African rural areas, which are marked by poverty, low level of education and poor health services. In order to further describe the rural area, it is important to examine some defining features.

Table 8.1 Urban/rural division of countries for the years 2015 and 2025

Region/ country	Urban population 2015	Rural population 2015	% Urban 2015	Urban population 2025	Rural population 2025	% Urban 2025
World	3,957,285,013	3,367,497,212	54.0	4,705,773,576	3,377,639,183	58.2
Africa	471,602,315	694,636,991	40.4	658,813,697	809,158,830	44.9
East Africa	101,034,466	293,719,352	25.6	154,745,070	356,483,116	30.3
Middle Africa	63,060,945	80,231,666	44.0	90,975,784	94,605,223	49.0
North Africa	112,068,513	104,995,632	51.6	136,283,788	114,697,334	54.3
Southern Africa	37,813,255	23,532,453	61.6	43,318,068	22,191,215	66.1
West Africa	157,625,136	192,157,888	45.1	233,490,987	221,181,942	51.4

Source UN (2015) and GeoHive (2016)

8.2.1 Rural Cultures

Rural areas come with distinct rural cultures shaped by the socio-spatial environment. Rural culture signifies the "degree to which they adhere to characteristically rural values, traditions, and customs, versus those of urban life" (Slama, 2014, p. 9). Because of the influence of information and communication technologies (ICTs), such as mobile phones, television, Internet, radio media and social media, it is debatable whether a distinct rural culture still exists; ICTs have likely provided some influence to dilute the so-called rural cultures. Despite some level of urban-rural acculturation, however, the remoteness of many African rural areas both spatially and technologically, suggests it is still accurate to speak of a distinct rural culture. The rural areas have retained traditional (and pre-colonial) values. This implies that there are still substantial deep-rooted cultural practices in rural areas. Rural culture is a peculiar way of life developed in relation to local values and infrastructures. In most instances in Africa, there is low level of infrastructure in African rural communities. Even agricultural practices are still predominantly done with crude equipment.

Rural life is still associated with deep traditional value system with a sense of community, conservative ideas and religious values (Hoggart, 1987). It is often characterized with primary industries (where available), mainly agriculture and small-scale commercial activities. In Africa, trading in agricultural products is the dominant commercial activity mostly in periodic community markets. Hoggart (1987) and Cloke and Chris (1985) identified some important features of including mechanical solidarity, simple economy and monocultural economy, low division of labor among others. All these features form the basis of rural life, which herein described as rural culture, is distinct from urban culture with a diverse economy, a high level of bureaucracy, low level of social bond among others. In general, this differential culture is unique and could be a major issue of consideration in health-care including health-related policies and interventions.

8.2.2 Relative Homogeneity

A typical rural community is homogeneous. This is, however, not to imply that one rural area is identical to another. In contrast to urban areas that attract people from all walks of life, and are highly diverse. Big cities like Cairo, Luanda, Nairobi and Lagos are miniature of their respective countries consisting of all ethnic groups and international community. Lagos, for instance, is often described as accommodating to all groups in Nigeria—meaning that it belongs to Nigerian (irrespective of ethnic group) although located in southwestern Nigeria. The same cannot be said of a typical Maasai community in rural Kenya as the community will be predominantly dominated by that single ethnic group. In the case of a rural community, diversity is not prominent. Apart from the population composition, homogeneity also reflects the nature of work, dress, customs, recreation, and orientation.

In addition, Beggs, Haines, and Hurlbert (2010, p. 306) observed that "personal networks in rural settings contain ties of greater intensity." It is further observed that such social networks are based on "kinship and neighborhood solidarities rather than on friendship, are smaller, are denser, and have greater educational, race-ethnic, and religious homogeneity, but less age and gender homogeneity." Homogeneity is, therefore, a common feature because rural dwellers share space, which is relatively small accommodating relatively small population. Homogeneity holds some positive implications for population health. In terms of community health interventions, there is often less need to account for wide differences or peculiarities, which could occur among different groups.

8.2.3 Low Population Density

One defining characteristic of rural areas is their low population density. The population of a typical rural area starts from around a few hundreds to thousands. Rural areas are sparsely populated with scattered settlements, unlike the urban area where there is concentration of people within the same place (densely).

In recent times, rural-urban migration has been the major factor responsible for low population growth in rural areas. More and more people (especially youth) are moving to the urban areas in search of better opportunities, such as employment, housing, education, and recreation. The low population density is positive for community mobilization and participation in development projects and health-related interventions. But that the communities are scattered, sometime, means duplication of efforts.

It is important to note that the urban areas are gradually encroaching upon the rural land. Developmental projects can claim lands and displace people, and this may lead to increasing land-constrained farming systems and impact negatively on rural income. Unlike most rural settings, a study observed that Kenya is a relatively densely populated area, with 40% of its rural people residing on 5% of its rural land (Muyanga & Jayne, 2014). Displacement or encroachment impacts adversely on population health, for example displacement is associated with stress and certain unmet need In general, the inability to develop the rural setting in order to retain the rural population also leads to urban congestion, and leave aging population at the rural end.

8.2.4 Highly Agrarian

Agriculture is the major occupation of rural populations all over the world. Rural areas are dominated by primary industries. In Africa, most rural dwellers are farmers, and in most instances, small scale farmers who still operate farming with little or no mechanization. In many African countries, due to other competitive enterprises, there has been a gradual reduction in public expenditure on agriculture over the years. Only in recent times, has there been a new drive to revive the agricultural sector, although the expenditure is still not commensurate with the requirements. Low investment in agriculture means low productive capacity for rural dwellers who depend fully on agriculture. Nigeria, for instance, moved from an agriculture-based economy to crude oil, which led to the gradual neglect of the agricultural sector. Only recently, especially because of the dwindling oil revenue, has there been a clamor for the government to diversify the economy and for people to return to agriculture.

In Tanzania, 80% of the population live and earn their living in rural areas, with agriculture as the primary means of livelihood. Although Tanzanian agriculture is dominated by small-scale (or subsistence) farming, agriculture accounts for a substantial portion of the GDP in Tanzania. The implication of large populations depending on agriculture is that any government investment in agriculture can strongly impact economic growth and cushion hunger crises. KIT (Royal Tropical Institute) (2005) observed that agriculture and rural development are gradually returning to international development agendas as a means of alleviating poverty and fostering broad-based and pro-poor economic development in countries where more than half of the population still depend on agriculture. In that same vein, many community-based health insurance schemes are targeted towards farmers (Ejughemre, 2014) and should consider rural occupation in health interventions.

8.2.5 Rural Poverty

Poverty is higher in rural than in urban areas. KIT (2005) observed that 75% of the poor live in the rural areas, and are desperately seeking ways to improve their living conditions and income. Rural poverty is often reproduced in each generation, due to perpetual deprivation of development projects. This is why Tekeuchi (2016) averred that the development issue in African rural areas has the same significance as before. The majority of African rural areas lack essentials amenities, such as electricity, water, health facilities and schools. Especially due to low literacy rates, rural populations have little capacity to improve their livelihood.

8.3 The State of Rural Health in Africa

Poverty is a fundamental determinant of health. It is a truism to correlate the high rate of poverty in rural areas to the high disease burden of (preventable) diseases. This huge disease burden is further increased by the deficient health services in rural areas. In addition, rural dwellers have low coverage of health insurance. Thus, poverty, a lack of health services and low insurance coverage exacerbates the healthcare situation in African rural areas.

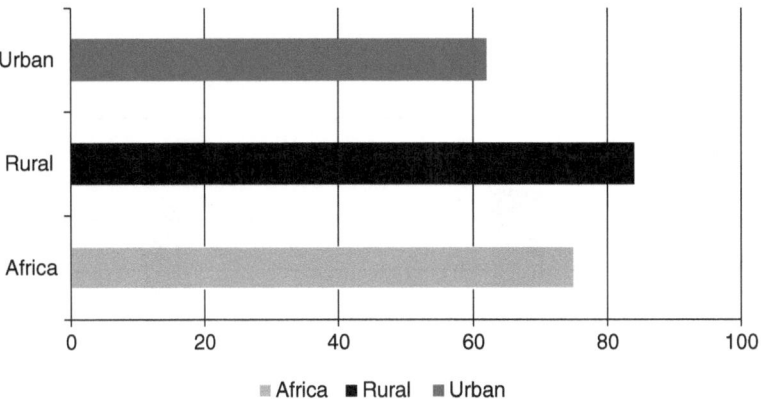

Fig. 8.1 Proportion of the rural population in Africa not protected by legislation or affiliated to a national health service or scheme, 2015 (percentages). *Source* Scheil-Adlung/ILO (2015)

The health status of those living rural areas is worse than in urban areas. As indicated in Table 8.1, up to 60% of the African population lives in rural areas but they are underserved with health services. While a high percentage of the African population has difficulties in accessing healthcare, the rural dwellers experience the worst effects. Scheil-Adlung/ILO (2015) observed that while up to 38% of global populations are without rights-based health coverage, global rural coverage is 2.5 times less than coverage in urban areas. In Africa, 83% of the rural population (see Fig. 8.1) has no entitlement to healthcare compared to 54% in Asia and the Pacific (Scheil-Adlung/ILO, 2015). The situation in Africa is a tragic because it shows that ensuring healthcare for all is a low priority for the government. Hence, all the health indicators from the rural areas are typically worse than those of their urban counterparts. As a consequence, the majority of rural dwellers (mostly poor) rely on public health institutions (where available) for healthcare. Unfortunately, the rural areas are underserved with health facilities.

Figures 8.1 and 8.2 show some information regarding the state of access to healthcare. While the problem of access also features in the urban setting, the alarming disparity can be observed when the large population size residing in the rural areas is considered. In many African countries, the rural population is very high. For instance, in countries such as Burundi, Ethiopia, Malawi, South Sudan, Uganda and Niger, up to 80% of the population lives in rural areas, while Eritrea, Chad, Lesotho, Swaziland and Burkina Faso have up to 70% residing in rural areas (GeoHive, 2016). Also in terms of access to health services, the financial burden is very high in the rural areas. Figure 8.2 shows some data across the world regions about rural populations without health coverage due to lack of financial resources.

The public health system in Africa is still highly unfavorable to the rural dwellers. Hence, the basic health indicators (regarding the most essential healthcare needs) are poor. In South Africa, Versteeg, Toit, and Couper (2013) submitted that rural communities are among the most disadvantaged in terms of access to

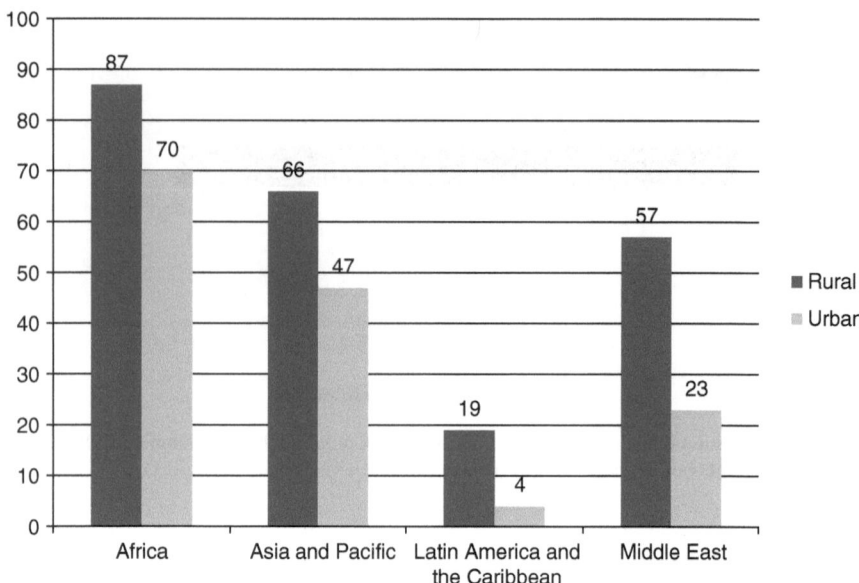

Fig. 8.2 Estimated health coverage gap due to financial deficits in rural/urban areas, selected regions, 2015 (percentages). *Source* Scheil-Adlung/ILO (2015)

quality healthcare; a child living in rural area is more than twice as likely to die in his/her first year of life as a child in an urban area. The same goes for various health conditions. For instance, in the face of lack of health workers, emergency cases involving severe bleeding and other severe conditions could lead to death. This is why there has been pressing global call to initiate rural health policies in Africa and around the world. This informed the introduction of a rural health strategy in Australia in 1994 rural proofing in the UK and a rural health mission in India (Versteeg et al., 2013). There must be "rural sensitivity" in health policy in a way that will examine differential policy impacts in rural area, and then efforts made to counter any adverse impact.

Even without the disease-specific incidence rate, the grand depiction is that of grossly inadequate coverage in rural areas compared to urban centers. This is one of the (sometimes-) neglected intra-country health disparities in access to health-care services. The extreme cases are reflected in those communities that have no health facility within 5-km reach and no mobile health services. This is a scenario of absolute deficiency of modern healthcare. Such communities rely on traditional medicine and forms of informal care which most times do not adequately meet health needs of community members. This is why the health indicators in African countries and rural areas in particular are poor. Beyond this general demographic representation of health in rural areas (in Figs. 8.1 and 8.2), it is important to examine some specific issues accounting for the rural-urban health disparities (with an emphasis on rural areas) of Africa.

8.4 Critical Healthcare Delivery Issues in Rural Communities

The poor healthcare services and health outcomes can be situated within certain issues? A grand tour of African rural areas is usually a testimony to the urban bias and series of relative deprivations, which account for poor rural health condition. Some of the critical healthcare delivery issues will be examined.

8.4.1 Facility Shortage

The first major healthcare challenge in rural areas is about availability of healthcare facilities. The distribution of health facilities between rural and urban areas is uneven, with the rural areas bearing the deficiency. Public health institutions usually serve the rural areas, as private providers often prefer highly populated areas (with potentially high-paying clients). A deficient infrastructure and extensive poverty in rural areas contributes to the shortage of healthcare facilities. A critical issue in healthcare access is the availability of a physical structure (even a mobile one). It has been generally recommended that individuals should not need to travel more than 5 km or 30 min to access healthcare services. But because of general spatial inequity in the distribution of health facilities, many rural residents must travel farther and/or longer to access healthcare.

Explaining spatial inequality in the distribution of health facilities in Pakistan, Zaidi (1985) examined the maldistribution of health facilities and observed that the health sector has grown primarily in response to the needs of the bourgeois (predominantly urban) classes. He highlighted two major reasons for maldistribution: the type of medical education in Pakistan, and the role of the government. Medical education is urban-biased and -based, hospital-oriented and uses a curative-care model. The government often invests heavily in urban areas at the expense of the rural population. Zaidi (1985) explained that the urban bias in distribution of health facility is a reflection of capitalist class structure, thus underlining that Pakistan's healthcare reflects political and economic expediency at the expense of the need principle. Thinking about the African scenario, Zaidi's observations are relevant. African governments play important roles in the allocation of health resources and determine where health facilities are located. The distribution of infrastructure is a reflection of governmental priorities, which may put some segments at a disadvantage. And truly, medical education is still elitist, that is why rural postings are not attractive. Dussault and Franceschini (2006) reiterated that there is always the drive towards modernization and industrialization to concentrate investments in urban areas, despite that a larger rural population. The drive resulted in an urban bias, and subsequent concentration of medical schools and health facilities in urban areas (Dussault & Franceschini, 2006). Therefore, ensuring a sufficient number of well-equipped health facilities is the first major step in extending health coverage to the rural population.

8.4.2   Shortage of Health Workers and Equipment in Rural Areas

While there is general shortage of health workers in Africa, the shortage in rural areas is more acute. For instance, Scheil-Adlung/ILO (2015) examined the coverage gap due to the health professional staff deficit in Nigeria and Zambia (with a threshold of 41.1 physicians, nurses and midwives per 10,000 population). The study indicated that the national average (of health professional staff) for Nigeria and Zambia were 60% and 81% deficits, respectively, but the rural-urban disparities were notable, with an urban/rural deficit of 37%/82% in Nigeria and 68%/89% in Zambia. In Tanzania, the national average is 3.5 doctors per 100,000 people. However,52% of all doctors work in the capital city, Dar es Salaam, giving it an average of 25 doctors per 100,000 people, compared to most rural areas which have one or less doctor per 100,000 (Kwesigabo et al., 2008).

Most advanced countries face the issue of maldistribution of health workers between urban and rural areas. For instance in the USA, the distribution of physicians remains skewed toward urban areas: rural America has 20% of the nation's population, but less than 11% of its physicians (Rickette, 2000). It was further observed that many rural communities continue to experience shortages of physicians, earning them the dubious title of Health Professional Shortage Areas (HPSAs) (Petterson, Phillips, Bazemore, & Koinis, 2013; Rickette, 2000). In the USA, the availability of primary healthcare physician in urban areas is more than the estimated requirement of 80/100,000 population while that of rural area is 68/100,000 (Petterson et al. 2013). At the global level, ILO estimated a 10.3-million health worker deficit with 70% deficits in rural areas.

In Africa, urban healthcare facilities are relatively better off than rural, in terms of equipment that facilitate health delivery. In most African countries, the general policy is to offer PHC in rural areas, with services commensurate to needs. Although PHC does not generally require sophisticated machinery, the basic equipment required is often unavailable. Kwesigabo et al. (2008) commented that "lack of equipment and unreliability of supplies (including vaccines, antibiotics, and other essentials) has been a major factor militating against the retention of health staff in rural areas." The chronic shortage of both staff and equipment in rural areas is a reality in Africa.

8.4.3   Poor Working Conditions and Infrastructure

Working conditions in rural areas, including remuneration, incentives and physical environment are relatively poor. It has been observed that one of the most "damaging effects of severely weakened and under-resourced health systems is the difficulty they face in producing, recruiting, and retaining health professionals" in rural areas (Lehmann, Dieleman, & Martineau, 2008). Poor working conditions have been repeatedly implicated in the flight of healthcare personnel from remote areas (Lehmann et al. 2008).

A majority of rural areas in Africa are riddled with deficient infrastructures, which make them very unattractive to health professionals to work and live in. The reasons for rural-urban migration include the search for better housing, education, and other essential services. The search for these services, which are usually deficient in rural areas, might explain poor retention of health workers in rural areas. Mensah (2002) and Ageyi-Baffour, Rominski, Nakua, Gyakobo, and Lori (2013) reiterated this issue when they explained that living conditions, including staff accommodation, schools and qualified teachers, good drinking water, reliable electricity, roads and transport, are important issues in the consideration of health workers' decision to accept or reject rural posting in Ghana (see also Lehmann et al., 2008).

Where there is limited or no electricity, it adversely affects the quality of health delivery, as most equipment requires power supply to function. The work and living environments are also negatively affected by lack of electricity. Where the roads are not good, it holds negative implication for referrals and access by patients within the neighborhoods. In general, the lack of infrastructure itself is a determinant of health, in this case, with negative outcomes, which might put pressure on available health facilities. Lack of potable water can increase the risk of water-borne diseases (Nwabor, Nnamonu, Martins, & Ani, 2016). This poor infrastructure is a part of most rural areas, and push workers to the urban areas where there are relatively better infrastructures.

8.4.4   Deep-Rooted Cultural Practices

Another critical issues relating to healthcare access in rural areas is deep-rooted cultural practices, which can contribute to high disease vulnerability in rural areas. While there are strengths relating to health in rural areas, such as high rate of social capital and strong social conscience, there are some embedded downsides that are detrimental to rural health. As it has been previous explained (Sect. 8.2.1), rural culture is still highly traditional, sometimes untouched of modern traits. This explains the high rate of cultural discriminatory and harmful practices in rural compared to urban areas. First, there is still the issue of acceptability of modern medicine in rural areas of Africa. One of the reasons contributing to this low acceptability is that most rural communities are underserved and have little knowledge of the efficacy of modern medicine. As previously observed (see Sect. 1.3.2), socio-cultural and religious norms affect acceptability of healthcare. This is why it is advocated that taking local values and health-related concepts into account are important in promoting healthcare acceptability. The important concern is that traditional cultural norms are stronger in rural areas.

Dillip et al. (2012) explained that social acceptability is relevant in studying illness perception, which is sometimes not coherent with biomedical notions, specifically in rural societies. They concluded that understanding local understanding/ knowledge, including health-related practices, is fundamental to ensuring acceptability of (modern) healthcare services, including disease control. Therefore, there is still a fundamental problem of weak (modern) healthcare alliances with rural populations, not only in terms of inadequate facilities and health workers, but also health-related beliefs.

Another dimension of the deep-rooted socio-cultural context is cultural practices, some of which are harmful to health. Most of the harmful cultural practices previously mentioned, such as FGM, early marriage and cleansing rituals, among others (see Sects. 2.5.2 and 5.3.3) are more prevalent in rural areas. For instance, in many rural societies, FGM is perceived as the physical proof confirming a girl's initiation through a rite of passage to adulthood and confirming her femininity and membership to the community (Kaplan, Hechavarría, Bernal, & Bonhoure, 2013) without considering the adverse socio-medical consequences (including urinary, vaginal and sexual problems, and psychological issues). Gender inequality is also stronger in rural areas, with more intense consequences. Many of the harmful cultural practices continue because they are often perceived as normal cultural trajectories. Therefore, the rural areas are still confronted with issues of social acceptability (as a dimension of access to healthcare) and culturally patterned vulnerability.

8.4.5 High Costs of Healthcare

As previously observed, poverty is higher in the rural areas (see Sect. 8.2.5). For rural populations, healthcare comes with high costs, both direct and indirect. In general, rural dwellers are often over-burdened with out-of-pocket payments, which do not guarantee financial protection. Most African countries are still battling on how to extend health insurance to the rural poor (see Sect. 4.3.1). In the meantime, most rural dwellers have to make direct payment to cover healthcare costs. Indirect costs of health include associated costs such as transportation fare and absenteeism from work/farming. Time used in travelling and waiting for healthcare could be re-directed to productive and income-generating activities. Rural dwellers often travel far to access healthcare because of limited number of health facilities.

A recent study by Matovu, Nanyiti, and Rutebemberwa (2014) examined costs related to malaria treatment in Uganda. The study found that rural households travelled for a significantly longer time to reach healthcare facilities and spent more time waiting (up to five times) than their urban counterparts. The implication is that, where healthcare is available, high cost is still a major barrier to accessing healthcare in rural areas in Africa. In situations where free primary healthcare is provided, the indirect costs might still impose some limitations (Goudge, Gilson, Russell, Gumede, & Mills, 2009). This is why Goudge et al. (2009) recommended more outreach services, and that fee removal should be accompanied by wider measures to ensure improved access.

8.5 Improving Access to Healthcare in Rural Areas

Improving healthcare coverage of rural populations is still a major challenge in Africa. The main barrier has been the lack of a strong political will to implement best practices, and prioritize and implement strategies that yield results. Since healthcare is a right, the practice of treating provision of healthcare services to rural areas in the form of charity (and in form of foreign aid) cannot be sustained. With strong political will and actions, African governments and health practitioners can move beyond mere "wishful thinking and efforts." There have been several workable recommendations based on empirical evidence.

In general, as previously mentioned, rural communities do not need healthcare facilities with a very high level of sophistication. They need primary healthcare that provides essential needs, social acceptable, with commensurate and sustainable technology. There must be functional referral system, for situations where advanced care is required. Many African countries have already launched a primary healthcare policy to cater to the essential needs of their citizens. The primary healthcare is embedded with principles that should make it effective but the high disease burden suggest that there are still badgering questions regarding implementation. Anyway, the underlying and critical matters are *strong political will and efficient use of available resources*. With the critical matters in mind, it is pertinent to reiterate three vital measures that can serve to enhance the health of the rural populace.

8.5.1 Essential Services/Infrastructures

As earlier observed, the rural areas are fraught with deficient infrastructures including health services, water and electricity supply, road networks, basic sanitation, educational facilities among others. These are vital amenities that can enhance development and decent living. The grossly inadequate of infrastructure is part of the reasons why health workers are hardly attracted to the rural areas. It is one of the issues explaining high disease vulnerability in rural areas. It is the part of the push factors in migration. And in context, these social amenities are strong correlates of health in many ramifications. With all these, provision of infrastructures will turn around the health plight in most rural areas. A strong commitment to rural development is a panacea to alleviating the suffering of the rural dwellers and enhancing improved health condition. The first major step is to ensure that services are available, in terms of the physical structure, manpower and equipment. Therefore, it is important that the government invest on infrastructural development including building of health facilities in rural areas.

8.5.2 Social Mobilization

Social mobilization is a major component of the primary healthcare system. It involves community participation. The ultimate objectives are to ensure self-reliance, self-determination and sustainability. Once community members are carried along in matters affecting them, they are empowered to take appropriate action. WHO (1997) observed "that social mobilization ensure that healthcare programs are sustainable through sound financing schemes, it promotes integration of healthcare in accordance with community priorities and helps to bridge the gap between community and health services." This will help to improve social acceptability and, subsequently, improve healthcare utilization.

Community health workers (CHWs) are important links in this respect, with the mandate to mobilize the community for health promotion and protection. This indicates that healthcare does not have to be curative services all round. Community mobilization also helps to raise awareness of health issues at the community level, including socio-cultural issues relating to population health. There is an imperative need for more outreach services meant for health promotion and disease prevention through outreach programs, the CHWs would be able to address barriers to care and explore community participation structures that can enhance population health (see Nxumalo, Goudge, & Thomas, 2013).

8.5.3   Extension of Community-Based Health Insurance (CBHI)

In order to ensure, financial protection and gradual abolition of out-of-pocket payment, there is need to invest in the coverage of CBHI to the rural dwellers in Africa (see also Sect. 4.3.1). Many communities are already benefitting from CBHI, especially in low- and middle-income countries. It is important that the program is intensified to ensure wider coverage. A systematic review of studies in African and Asia indicated strong evidence that CBHI improves service utilization and protects members financially, by reducing their out-of-pocket expenditure, and that CBHI improves resource mobilization (Spann et al., 2012). The study concluded that CBHI offers some protection against the detrimental effects of user fees and a promising avenue towards universal healthcare coverage.

References

Ageyi-Baffour, P., Rominski, S., Nakua, E., Gyakobo, M., Lori, J. R. (2013). Factors that influence midwifery students in Ghana when deciding where to practice: a discrete choice experiment. *BMC Medical Education, 13*, 64. doi:10.1186/1472-6920-13-64.

Beggs, J. J., Haines, V. A., Hurlbert, J. S. (2010). Revisiting the rural-urban contrast: personal networks in nonmetropolitan and metropolitan settings. *Rural Sociology, 61*(2), 306–325.

Cloke, P., & Chris, P. (1985). *Rural resource management.* London: Croom Helm.

Dala-Clayton, B., Dent, D., Dubois, O. (2013). *Rural planning in developing countries: supporting natural resource management and sustainable livelihoods.* London: Earthscan.

Dillip, A., Alba, S., Mshana, C., Hetzel, M. W., Lengeler, C., Mayumana, I., et al. (2012). Acceptability—a neglected dimension of access to healthcare: findings from a study on childhood convulsions in rural Tanzania. *BMC Health Services Research, 12*, 113. doi:10.1186/1472-6963-12-113.

Dussault, G., & Franceschini, M. C. (2006). Not enough there, too many here: understanding geographical imbalances in the distribution of the health workforce. *Human Resources for Health, 4*, 12. doi:10.1186/1478-4491-4-12.

Ejughemre, U. J. (2014). Scaling-up health insurance through community-based health insurance schemes in rural sub-Saharan African communities. *Journal of Hospital Administration, 3*(1), 14–22.

GeoHive. (2016). Urban/rural division of countries for the years 2015 and 2025. http://www.geohive.com/earth/pop_urban.aspx. Accessed 11 July 2016.

Goudge, J., Gilson, L., Russell, S., Gumede, T., Mills, A. (2009). The household costs of health care in rural South Africa with free public primary care and hospital exemptions for the poor. *Tropical Medicine and International Health, 14*(4), 458–467.

Hoggart, K. (1987). *Rural development: a geographical perspective*. New York: Croom Helm.

Kaplan, A., Hechavarría, S., Bernal, M., Bonhoure, I. (2013). Knowledge, attitudes and practices of female genital mutilation/cutting among health care professionals in The Gambia: a multiethnic study. *BMC Public Health, 13*, 851. doi:10.1186/1471-2458-13-851.

KIT (Royal Tropical Institute). (2005). Rural development in sub-Saharan Africa: policy perspectives for agriculture, sustainable resource management and poverty reduction. *Bulletins of the Royal Tropical Institute* 370, Amsterdam: Royal Tropical Institute (KIT).

Kwesigabo, G., Mwangu, M. A., Kakoko, D. C., Warriner, I., Mkony, C. A., Killewo, J., et al. (2008). Tanzania's health system and workforce crisis. *Journal of Public Health Policy, 33*, S35–S44. doi:10.1057/jphp.2012.55.

Lehmann, U., Dieleman, M., Martineau, T. (2008). Staffing remote rural areas in middle- and low-income countries: a literature review of attraction and retention. *BMC Health Services Research, 8*, 19. doi:10.1186/1472-6963-8-19.

Matovu, F., Nanyiti, A., Rutebemberwa, E. (2014). Household health care-seeking costs: experiences from a randomized, controlled trial of community based malaria and pneumonia treatment among under-fives in eastern Uganda. *Malaria Journal, 13*, 222. doi:10.1186/1475-2875-13-222.

Mensah, K. (2002). *Attracting and retaining health staff: a critical analysis of the factors influencing the retention of health workers in deprived/hardship areas*. Accra: Yak-Aky Services.

Muyanga, M., & Jayne, T. S. (2014). Effects of rising rural population density on smallholder agriculture in Kenya. *Food Policy, 48*, 98–113.

Nwabor, F. O., Nnamonu, E. I., Martins, P. E., Ani, O. C. (2016). Water and waterborne diseases: a review. *International Journal of Tropical Diseases & Health, 12*(4), 1–14.

Nxumalo, N., Goudge, J., Thomas, L. (2013). Outreach services to improve access to health care in South Africa: lessons from three community health worker programmes. *Global Health Action, 6*, doi:10.3402/gha.v6i0.19283.

Petterson, S. M., Phillips, R. L., Bazemore, A. W., Koinis, G. T. (2013). Unequal distribution of the U.S. primary care workforce. *American Family Physician, 87*(11), online.

Rickette, T. C. (2000). Health care in rural communities: the imbalance of health care resource distribution needs correction. *Western Journal of Medicine, 173*, 294–295.

Scheil-Adlung, X., & ILO. (2015). Global evidence on inequities in rural health protection: new data on rural deficits in health coverage for 174 countries. *International Labour Office, Social Protection Department*, Geneva: ILO (Extension of Social Security series; No 47).

Slama, K. M. (2014). Rural culture is a diversity issue. *Minnesota Psychologist*, pp. 9–13.

Spann, E., Mathijssen, J., Tromp, N., McBain, F., Have, A., Baltussen, R. (2012). The impact of health insurance in Africa and Asia: a systematic review. *Bulletin of the World Health Organization, 90*(9), 685–692.

Tekeuchi, S. (2016). African studies and rural development. http://www.ide.go.jp/English/Publish/Download/Workshop/pdf/02_01.pdf. Accessed 13 July 2016.

UN. [United Nations, Department of Economic and Social Affairs, Population Division] (2015). World urbanization prospects: the 2014 Revision, ST/ESA/SER.A/366.

Versteeg, M., Toit, L., Couper, I. (2013). Building consensus on key priorities for rural health care in South Africa using the Delphi technique. *Global Health Action*, *6*, 19522. doi:10.3402/gha.v6i0.19522.

WHO [World Health Organization]. (1997). Mobilization of the community in support of health for all. Technical Paper, Regional Committee for the Eastern Mediterranean, Nasr City, Cairo: WHO.

Zaidi, A. S. (1985). The urban bias in health facilities in Pakistan. *Social Science and Medicine*, *20*(5), 473–482.

Chapter 9
Pastoral Nomadism and Health in Africa

9.1 Introduction

The pastoral nomads constitute a distinct category of people, both in Africa and around the world. The situation in Africa is a bit peculiar because of the distinct and differential circumstances. In health discourse, pastoral nomads have been neglected, historically. And because of their way of life, they are important public health category, and in sociology, a sociological group. Because of their geographic isolation from even rural areas (in Africa, they often reside in the deep forest), their lack of access to basic life necessities, especially in their modern forms, is more intense than other groups. It is sometimes, wondered why they have not been categorized as a distinct vulnerable population, especially in Africa.

This chapter will look at various health-related issues among the pastoralists, with special focus on the nomadic pastoralists. Because of their nomadic nature, they are not bound to one particular geographic area in Africa. This decentralization makes it difficult for healthcare professionals to (know how to) meet their healthcare needs.

A student once asked: there are still many settlements underserved with healthcare, some without any health facility in Africa, why do we have to run after the pastoral nomads with healthcare? The answer to this question lies in a number of reasons.

1. The right to health is a fundamental human right of every individual (see Sect. 2.2). Healthcare has to be tailored to the needs of the clients in a way that it will be accessible. Disregarding their healthcare needs is an infraction of their fundamental human rights. It is a collective responsibility to respect their peculiar pastoral way of life, which is indeed a productive activity for the community in general.
2. Some of the fundamental principles governing healthcare are universalism and equality. Universal coverage implies that everyone is covered, irrespective of his or her personal or social circumstances (see Sect. 1.4). Nomadic pastoralists are geographically and socially marginalized (Zinsstag, Taleb, & Craig, 2006) and therefore a vulnerable population. Any exclusive principle regarding their health needs will intensely reinforce their vulnerability.

© Springer International Publishing AG 2018   125
J. Amzat, O. Razum, *Towards a Sociology of Health Discourse in Africa*,
DOI 10.1007/978-3-319-61672-8_9

3. That they are mobile is a vital reason to ensure their adequate healthcare coverage. As it will later be examined (see Sect. 8.4.3), mobility or migration is a major factor in population health because it facilitates human contacts. In cases of infectious diseases, a mobile population serves as carrier in the transmission of diseases. What affects a mobile community might very quickly become a national or even global emergency.

4. The concept of "One health" or medicine is also applicable to situation of the nomadic pastoralists. "One health" signifies that the health of humans is connected with the health of animals and the environment. Not only is healthcare required by the pastoralists, the animals also require veterinary services. Substantial milk and meat that the general population consumes are sourced from the animals that the pastoralists preserve. Such products must be safe for human consumption. And more importantly, there is often transmission of (zoonotic) diseases from animals to humans (see Sect. 8.4.1). There must be integrative care systems to ensure mutual health for both humans and animals to avert any adverse consequences on global health.

Following the background, the chapter will start by looking at some conceptual definitions, then nomadic life and disease vulnerability, and some guiding principles for effective health coverage of the nomadic communities.

9.2   Some Conceptual Clarifications

It is important to define some relevant concepts, which will enhance some understanding. Concepts that will be examined include pastoralism, nomadism, transhumans and sedentarism.

9.2.1   Pastoralism

Pastoralism simply implies the raising of livestock on "natural" pasture, unimproved by human intervention (Salzman, 2004), i.e., pasture not cultivated or tended by people. The raising of animals is done on open fields and routes, a kind of free grazing, in most parts of the world, and in Africa in particular. The animals, often domesticated by the pastoralists, include cattle, goats, camels, sheep and horses, among others. Pastoralism can be defined as an "economic and social system well adapted to dryland conditions and characterized by a complex set of practices and knowledge that has permitted the maintenance of a sustainable equilibrium among pastures, livestock and people" (Rota & Sperandini, 2009). For some precision, Rota and Sperandini (2009) further observed that pastoralists are people who derive more than 50% of their income from livestock and livestock products, while agropastoralists are people who derive less than 50% of their income from livestock and livestock products, and most of the remaining income from cultivation. The central issue is the dependence on livestock as a social passion and means of earnings. This precision differentiates pastoralists from mere animal domestication or farmers who also domesticate one or two animals. The agricultural focus of the pastoralist is livestock, with some living entirely from the livestock.

It can be noted from the definition that there is an intricate triangular relationship of people, livestock and pasture. The pastoralists enter into mutually supportive relationships with their herds and into a dependent or parasitic relations with the natural environment of their eco-system. Man and herds live in a symbiotic community (IESS, 2008). The livelihood of the people depends on the livestock that they rear, which constitute their economic possession or means of earning. To sustain the livestock, pasture is needed; the pasture is the main food for the livestock. The pasture is sometimes scarce because pastoralists mostly reside on dry lands, or there is seasonal scarcity between the rain and dry seasons. This is why it is a task to sustain the livestock, with pastures and water. The scarce resources are the major determinants of pastoral social organization and general patterns of livelihood, which can be influenced by the needs of the livestock.

The pastoralists along with their animals, live mainly in dry and remote areas. Pastoralism is, therefore, a fulltime agroeconomic activity. It has been observed that the livelihood of the pastoralists depends on their intimate knowledge of the surrounding ecosystem and on the well-being of their livestock. This is why it was observed that pastoralism functions as a cultural system with a characteristic ecology (IESS, 2008). Due to the ecological requisite to survival of both the pastoralists and the animals, the pastoralist community is an ecological unit. Because of the distinct sociocultural patterns and adaptation, the social group is also a sociocultural community (IESS, 2008). What is noteworthy is that, based on the knowledge of the ecosystem, movement can be initiated to search for abundant pasture and water. This shift in residence and location is a major feature of the pastoralists in Africa. The pastoralists can be very nomadic! Pastoralism is connected with nomadism, transhumance and sedentarism (Muhammad-Baba and Amzat, 2012).

9.2.2 Nomadism, Transhumance and Sedentarism

Nomadism in this sense is pastoral nomadism, which is an adaptive process or response in the management of livestock involving movement in search of needs of the livestock and the pastoralists, usually necessitated by ecological factors. Technically, pastoral nomadism is a "complex set of practices and knowledge that has permitted the long-term maintenance of a sophisticated 'triangle of sustainability' that includes plants, animals, and people" (Koocheki & Gliessman, 2005, p. 113). Specifically, Muhammad-Baba and Amzat (2012, p. 78) observed that "it is possible for a specific area to be overgrazed and water unavailable in certain periods…", "… necessitating movement of flocks and herds in response to pasture needs and other factors such as water, temperature, disease and predators"—this is called pastoral nomadism.

The pastoral nomads are always on the move in search of green pastures and water for their livestock. In this regard, mobility is a major strategy for exploiting scarce resources in order to maintain the triangle of sustainability. Hence the movement is often cyclical and periodical. The extent of the movement is limitless in terms of distance; it generally depends on the availability of sustainable resources. The movement could range from a few kilometers to cross boarder movement. The movement might also be based on establishment of temporary or makeshift posts or residence, the stability of which is a function of the continuous availability of the said scarce resources. The movement could be cyclical, as some nomads might return to a focal site after some period of time, but a total shifting of residence is also possible. The movement is often on established routes sustained through the knowledge of the nomads about the availability of pasturage. Therefore, nomadic pastoralism is a lifestyle involving "residential mobility designed to obtain resources such as pasture for domestic herds, and access to market for the herds and their products" (Muhammad-Baba and Amzat, 2012, p. 78).

With relatively stable focal sites, pastoralists move in the direction of pasture and water during any seasons. The seasonal movement of nomadic pastoralist is called transhumance (Smith, 1992a). Transhumance is, therefore, a form of nomadism and pastoralism, expressed through a pattern of mostly seasonal movement. Transhumance is mostly practiced in those parts of the world where there are highlands or areas that are too cold to be inhabited and utilized for grazing except in summer (the seasonal movement is alternated between winter and summer). In many instances, seasonal movement might be undertaken by the herder, leaving the family behind.

After being nomadic for a period of time, some nomads become sedentary. Sedentarism (sometimes called sedentism) simply refers to the practice of living in one place for a relatively long time. Sedentarization "is the process of formerly nomadic populations settling into non-mobile communities, and applies to foraging populations, livestock keeping pastoralists, and other occupational or ethnic groups that were formerly mobile" (Fratkin, Roth, & Nathan, 2004, p. 532). Fratkin *et al.* (2004) observed that throughout the arid regions of Africa, formerly mobile pastoral populations are becoming sedentary. It is, therefore, not uncommon to observe many formally nomadic pastoral groups settling down in ecologically and economically strategic places. Fratkin *et al.* (2004) confirmed that some previously nomadic pastoral populations have settled near towns to market milk, meat, and livestock, as well as taken advantage of new opportunities in wage labor, education, and access to healthcare. The act of sedentism has been advocated as a major means of resolving some huge problems (drought and attacks) confronting nomadic pastoralists.

9.3   Nomadic Pastoralism in Africa

Nomadic pastoralism is a major type of pastoralism in Africa. At a period in time, was a change from hunting to domestication of animals. There are a number of factors responsible for the growth of pastoralism in Africa, including ecological, social and economic factors. For instance on the ecology, Smith (1992b, 2005) argued that, as the extensive grasslands of Africa with rainfall <500 mm (the tsetse boundary) offer limited opportunity for agriculture, they are optimal for pastoral activities. The development of nomadic pastoralism is attributed to the uneven availability of range and water across Africa. Hence, nomadic pastoralism developed as adaptation to the unpredictable natural ecology (Adriansen, 1997).

It is difficult to obtain specific estimates of the number of nomadic pastoralists in Africa; mobile African pastoralists are undercounted or excluded from many data sources because of the difficulties in enumerating mobile individuals (Randall, 2015). While most data available are speculative, there is no doubt that they constitute a significant number and should warrant attention of relevant nations and even at the global level. In sub-Saharan Africa, pastoral and agro-pastoral communities account for 20 million and 240 million individuals, respectively (Blench, 2001). The nomadic pastoralists can be found across several African states (see Box 9.1 for a non-exhaustive list). Also see Figs. 9.1 and 9.2 showing the Nuerland in Ethiopia. Kenya claims the most pastoral ethnic groups, including the Rendille, Maasai, Samburu, Pokot, and Gabra, among others. It should also be noted that not all people within each tribe are nomads. In Nigeria, there are many Fulanis who have long abandoned pastoralism for white-collar jobs. The same is true for the Maasai and other previously nomadic groups in Kenya and Tanzania.

Box 9.1 African nomadic pastoralists

Ababdeh	Egypt/Sudan
Afars	Ethiopia/Djibouti
Bejah	Sudan
Berbers	North Africa
Borana Oromo	Ethiopia/Kenya
Fulanis/Fulbe	West Africa
Gabra	Ethiopia/Kenya
Karamojong	Uganda/Kenya
Maasai	Kenya/Tanzania
Mrazig	Tunisia
Nuer	South Sudan/Ethiopia
Pokot	Kenya/Uganda
Rendille	Kenya
Sharawis	Morocco/Algeria
Somalis	Horn of Africa
Tuaregs	Niger/Mali
Toubou	Chad/Niger
Trekboers	South Africa

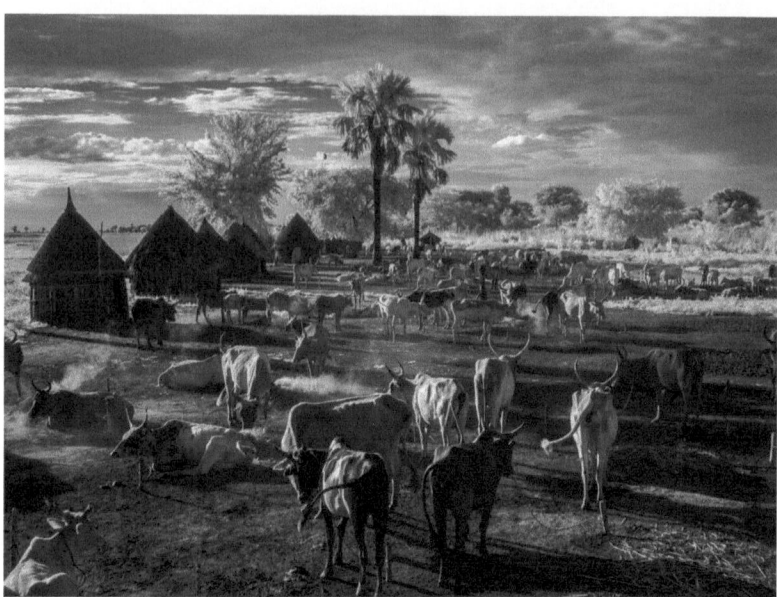

Fig. 9.1 Pastoralist huts in Nuerland Ethiopia. *Picture Credit* Steven Wade Adams (DVM, PhD)

The distinctive lifestyles, adaptive process and socio-economic activities of the nomads have significant implications for their wellbeing. The core strategies of the pastoralists are based on mobility, flexibility, efficiency and reserves. It should be acknowledeged that most pastoralists reside or move around in a patchy, unpredictable and low-productivity envoronment. They navigate their ways through rigorous adaptive processes to survive. This holds true not only for the adult members but also newborns and young persons.

Unlike in precolonial Africa, the adpative processes of the nomads have come under serious threat. Mobility has been curtailed due to expansion in agricultural practices, such as more land earmarked for cultivation on some on the pastoralist routes. More often than not, the (sedenetary) farmers because of relatively permanent residency, have upper claim over the pastoralists, on land and other vital resources. This has, in many instances, generated problems of encroachment. In a fair sense, based on historical antecedents, it is often difficult to judge enroachment, which has led to several thousand deaths and loss of property especially over the past 50 years. Farmer-pastoralist conflict is a major problem in areas where pastoralists are significant in number.

The nomadic pastoralists have also been confronted with boundary problems. Unlike in the precolonial era, where there were less boundary demarcations and restrictions, now immigration policies and boundary enforcement have not been favorable to the nomadic population. As previously mentioned, due to certain social changes and pressures, some previous nomads are now sedentary. The pastoralists are highly productive and responsible for the substantial supply of milk

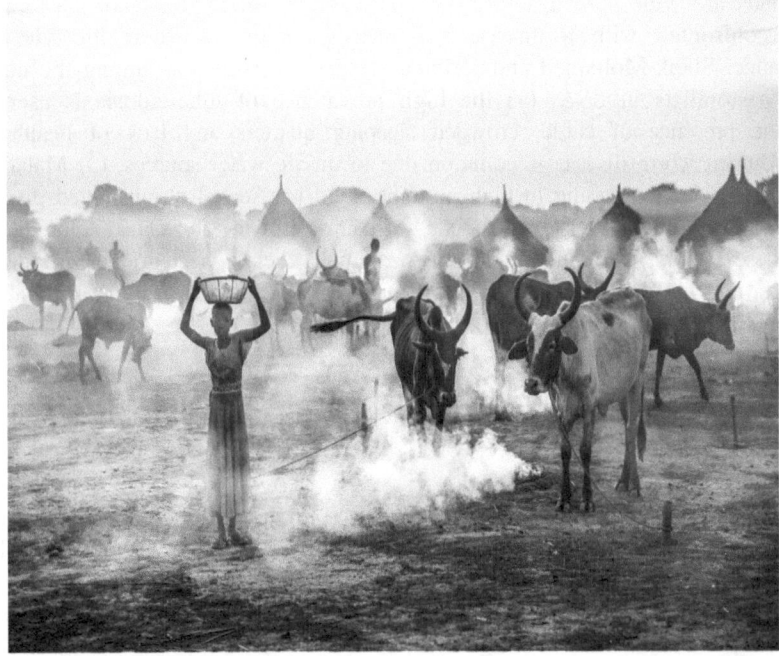

Fig. 9.2 Pastoralist huts of Nuerland (Ethiopia) also showing some young domestic workers. *Picture Credit* Steven Wade Adams (DVM, PhD)

and meat in Africa. In several African communities, there is significant dependence on pastoralists to provide certain basic needs such as milk and meat. Various types of livestock (sheep, goats, cattle, camels, yak, donkeys and horses) provide nutrition, transport, clothing and shelter (Zinsstag *et al.*, 2006). It is an important means of foreign exchange. Leathers obtained from livestock are sold all over the world, and for further processing into various materials for human use. Zinsstag *et al.* (2006) further observed that nomadic pastoralist livestock production contributes up to 15% of the GDP for a population estimated at <6% of the total population in Chad. In several other African countries, it is difficult to estimate the economic contribution of pastoralism because the pastoralists mostly operate within informal sector with very little formalization.

9.4 Pastoral Nomadic Life and Disease Vulnerability

Previous sections have stressed that the nomadic pastoralists have unique ways of life and adaptive strategies, which revolve around their herds. Importantly, their life demands and challenges are also connected with mobility; the pastoral nomads are wide spread across the continent of Africa. Nomadic pastoralists are confronted with a disease vulnerability unique to their lifestyle. For instance, Sheik-Mohamed and Velema (1999) observed that among the nomadic pastoralists in SSA, (1) the high prevalence of tuberculosis is ascribed to the presence of cattle, crowded sleeping quarters and lack of healthcare; (2) Guinea worm disease is common due to unsafe water sources; (3) Malaria is usually epidemic, leading to high mortality; and (4) Sexually transmitted diseases spread easily due to lack of treatment. A great deal of literature has explored some of these factors, including proximity to animals, dietary behavior, environmental issues, and limited access to essential amenities (see Swift, Toulmin & Chatting, 1990; Desta, 2016).

9.4.1   Proximity to Animals

Due to their extreme dependence on and close proximity to their animals, the pastoralists are at very high risk of exposure to animal diseases (zoonosis). This includes such parasites as echinococcosis, and infections such as brucellosis, bovine tuberculosis, anthrax and rabies, many of which are endemic to sub-Saharan Africa (Moritz, Ewing & Garabed, 2013). Many zoonotic infections are transmissible between humans and animals. Schelling (2002) observed that there are two major means of disease transmission between humans and animals: the direct mode involves contact with an infected animal, while the indirect mode is through contact with a vector.

Health problems among nomadic communities are not limited to zoonotic infections; tuberculosis, acute respiratory and gastrointestinal infections, vaccine preventable diseases, STI and parasitic infections are also found (Schelling *et al.*, 2010; Zinsstag *et al.*, 2006).

There is little or no specific data on morbidity and mortality rate among the nomadic population. Zoonotic diseases have the potential to seriously threaten human health and to lead to global public health concerns. For instance, in a comprehensive identification of 1415 species of infectious pathogens to humans, 868 (61%) are zoonotic, that is, transmissible between humans and animals (Taylor, Latham & Woolhouse, 2001). Out of the 175 pathogens considered to be emerging diseases, 75% are zoonotic. Exposure of a nomadic population to such pathogens could significantly aid the spread of such diseases, raising global public health concerns, such as the cases of severe acute respiratory syndrome (SARS) and avian flu. Unfortunately, the level of awareness about zoonosis is very poor, even in pastoral environments (see Desta, 2016). Thus, there is need for an integrative approach to the human-animal health link especially among the nomadic population to curtail transmission and spread of infectious disease.

9.4.2   Dietary Behavior

The major foods available to the pastoralists are livestock products. The pastoralists often depend on a diet rich in (mostly raw) milk and other uncooked animal products. Schelling (2002) reported that transmission of pathogens from livestock to pastoralists might occur, e.g., through consumption of uncooked milk or through animal obstetric work. It is not uncommon for pastoralists and other family members to suck raw milk direct from animal breasts and to drink blood obtained from slaughtering animals. Sometimes, animals are (sometimes) intentionally pierced to obtain raw blood for drinking (see Fig. 9.3). A study found that nomadic pastoralists often give blood, animal's milk and bitter herbs to infants below six months, which affects exclusive breastfeeding (Chege, Kimiywe, & Ndungu, 2015). Some of those animals might be diseased. There are many zoonotic foodborne diseases. Without the exception of milk, most foods are consumed without observing proper hygiene.

An empirical study (Chege *et al.*, 2015) documented the major dietary issues among children of the pastoralists of Kenya. They observed that, despite the abundance of animals belonging to the household, animal products remain inaccessible to most children. One explanation for this is that livestock are considered a sign of

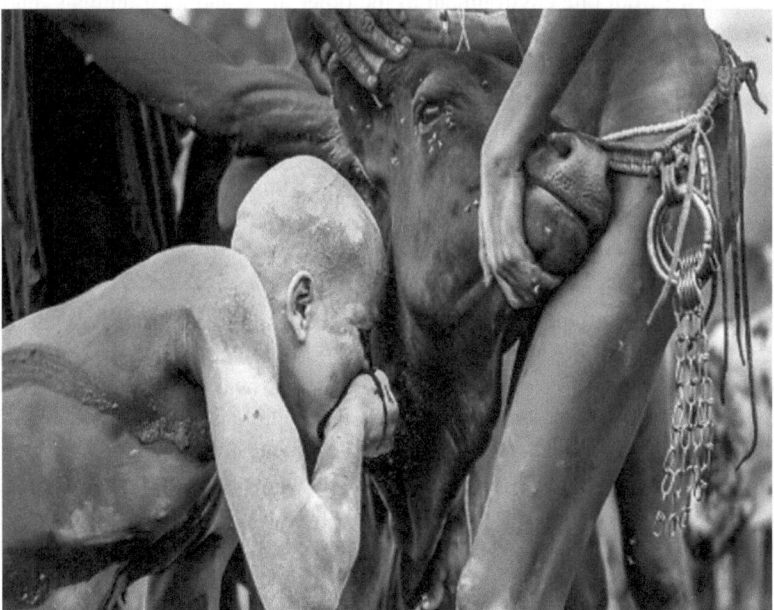

Fig. 9.3 Pastoralists pierced a cow to drink raw blood. *Picture Credit* Steven Wade Adams (DVM, PhD)

wealth, and therefore mainly slaughtered only on special occasions. Children were found to consume mainly cereals and legumes. Consumption of vegetables among the children is limited, since vegetables are perceived to be livestock feed. For most nomadic pastoralists, land is exclusively for grazing, not cultivation. This affects dietary intake, which may lack diversification: mostly cereals, legumes and milk all year round. For the nomads, there is little guarantee of an appropriately balanced diet, due to their mobile life that sometimes leads them to the Sahara desert of North Africa and other times to the rainforest of West Africa.

9.4.3 Mobility

As earlier observed, nomadism involves movement in search of some scare resources. Because of the growing land cultivation, their movements are patterned to avoid as much agricultural land as possible. This is why Zinsstag et al. (2006, p. 565) observed that "the nomadic way of life makes access to health dispensaries in villages difficult, as groups with animals have to avoid areas with crops, and visits to markets often exclude the most vulnerable – women and children." Randall (2010) observed that mobility could influence health through three principal pathways: changing susceptibility, exposure and quality of care. As the nomads move from one environment to the other, they and their animals might be exposed to new infections. Specifically, they are often exposed to new pathogens and natural hazards, including bites and stings from different creatures. The nomads might also be leaving behind some form of healthcare services without knowledge of another one nearby. The pastoralists might also be unable to access healthcare because of language barriers and a lack of knowledge of the health system in the new environment. In a study among the nomads in SSA, Sheik-Mohamed and Velema (1999) observed that existing healthcare systems are in the hands of settled populations and rarely benefit the nomads due to cultural, political and economic obstacles (see also Okeibuinor et al., 2013).

It is also difficult to maintain veterinary services for the animals that might reduce the risk of zoonosis. Mocellin and Foggin (2008) observed that the seasonal migration of pastoralists tends to increase the risk of poor health. Specifically, the study reported an inverse association between spatial mobility and health status among the herders. Conditions are often poorer among women and children. Especially for children, there might be low access to immunization services and other child healthcare. It has been observed that nomadic individuals generally have low immunization rates because their mobility renders immunization programs costly and logistically difficult, and health service provision is poor in remote areas (Randall, 2010). In cases where the children move with the family, they are particularly vulnerable in the face of intense temperate, due to their relatively low immunity.

Due to the high risk of zoonosis among the animals and the herders, contact populations might also be at risk. Long distance travel by the herders and animals often spread risk of zoonosis and other contagious diseases across regions. The contact population can also pose some risk to the pastoralists. Nomads often avoid epidemics such as measles by moving away from areas with health risks (Sheik-Mohamed and Velema, 1999). The pastoralists also need to avoid predators or defend themselves and the animals when they meet predators. One major consequence of this mobility is famer-pastoralist conflict, which can also be regarded as risk exposure. Annually, a significant number of deaths and property destruction are attributed to this conflict. Apart from adverse effects of nomadism on health, there could also be some benefits. A non-sedentary lifestyle often reduces risk of obesity and associated health conditions. In general, nomadism holds significant health implications.

9.4.4 Ecological Challenges

The arid and semi-arid rangelands are highly diverse in climate, land forms, soil types and vegetation, with characterized high spatial and temporal variability (Oba & Lusigi, 1987). Pastoral nomadism is one of the major means of adaptation to variable forage supplies and water distribution. Recurrent drought is a common problem in African rangelands, which adversely affect forage production and water availability (Oba & Lusigi, 1987). Pastoral nomads occupy the arid and semi-arid regions of SSA. They travel in the hot season of the Sahara with little or no safety measures. The nomads are also exposed to various weather conditions, and endure all the changes in environment throughout the year. They are exposed to hot, dry and dusty zones. Rearing animal in rangelands always exposes the pastoralists to sunlight, which is correlated with dehydration, heat cramps, heat exhaustion, heat stroke and skin cancer.

Loutan and Lamotte (1984) long ago observed that certain periods of the year are usually disastrous to the nomads. They observed that the end of the dry season (March to July) is usually critical for the Wodaabe herders. The period is fraught with high temperatures, lack of water and greater distances between camp and water, due to the increasingly scarce pasture. In search of water, the nomads often rely on dug wells. It is also strenuous drawing water for the animals. The period is also characterized with poor nutritional status due to complete reliance on millet, which is not sufficient for energy needs. The period also marks the end of the hot season. The wet season is also characterized with its own challenges, including cold.

Drought is usually a major disaster to the pastoralists and a major determinant of movement. It is often responsible for animal death. Therefore, nomads like to concentrate near water sources or even in relief camps, sometimes with grievous consequences for their health (Sheik-Mohamed and Velema, 1999). Apart from severe drought (or periods of unusual rainfall), wind and epidemics may also decimate the number of herds. The pastoralists are often aware, through their traditional means and adaptive patterns, of impending ecological challenge. It is not always an easy task to respond adequately especially in a manner that would not affect the herdsmen, household members and animals. The herdsmen rely on reserves and alliances with other pastoral households to survive disasters or ecological challenges, since there is hardly any formal support or safety nets from any quarters.

9.4.5 Socioeconomic and Cultural Practices

Like other African groups, the pastoral nomads have a unique culture shaped by pastoralism and nomadism. Some of the general structures are, however, reflections of the general culture. One fundamental aspect of the pastoralist way of life is "cattle complex",which is described as an extensive ritual usage of cattle with an emotional attachment to or identification with cattle (see Wurzinger, Ndumu, Okeyo & Sölkner, 2011). When the cattle are sick, the pastoralists are sick! The attachment with cattle is usually so intense that a common urban legend is that a typical pastoralist values the life of a herd over the life of other humans, even his children. Typically, pastoralists are generally regarded as poor and vulnerable. Their poverty is due to a number of factors including poor housing, poor diets, bad clothing and low household valuables. But considering their assets (cattle), the pastoralists are relatively better off when compared with the general poor population in Africa.

Among pastoralists, there is an entrenched gender division of labor. For instance, the adult males are usually in charge of decision-making regarding the household and herds, while the private sphere is mostly for women, involving taking care of the children, cooking, milking the cattle, and marketing of the dairy products. Men are often responsible for general care of the animals and for moving around with them. A substantial majority of pastoralists in West Africa are Muslims; this implies that they also follow some Islamic dictates. Over the years, the pastoralists have also developed distinct ethno-veterinary practices in the care of the animals, because a majority of them do not have access to modern veterinary services. All these issues affect the health status of the pastoral nomads.

The nomads have a number of traditional adaptive practices. For instance, the cow urine and dung are used for medicinal purposes, purification of the environment and other domestic uses. Hygiene standards are very poor, especially during dry season. Axweso (2011) observed that among the pastoralists in Tanzania during such season, baths are rarely taken, cloths are not washed and food utensils are only scraped clean from meal to meal. It is further observed that water points are usually shared with the herds and some critical water needs are met through cattle urine (Axweso, 2011). In another study, some cattle keepers mentioned the use of cattle urine mixed with milk and used as a laxative, and as detergent for cleaning milk pots (Wurzinger et al., 2011). In traditional medicine, urine-herb mix is used as a mouthwash or for treatment of skin infections. Some pastoralists also mentioned the use of (cattle) blood mixed with milk as a beverage for home consumption (Wurzinger *et al.*, 2011). The aforementioned traditional and adaptive practices have implications for health.

9.4.6 Limited Access to Essential Services

From the foregoing discussion, it is evident that pastoral nomads usually have very low access to basic facilities. Because they are always on the move, building infrastructures for them is usually a difficult task. This low access to essential services (such as water and power supply, sanitation, health services and education) is a major consequence of mobility. Hygiene and sanitation projects have generally been considered impossible, in view of pastoralists' lifestyle (Axweso, 2011) since they are very mobile. A majority of the pastoral nomads have no formal education, which may account for low levels of health literacy and an understanding of the health impacts of poor hygiene. Efforts to provide nomadic education in several African countries have only recorded partial success.

In general, Shiekh and Kwaak (2015) observed that health practices are influenced by the mobile lifestyle of nomads, their low level of education and knowledge, gender norms, beliefs, values and attitudes, and their geographical locations. As previously observed, the existing healthcare services are under the control of the settled communities and unfortunately, are ill-adapted to the nomadic lifestyle. Among the pastoralists, the major determinants of health are generally unfavorable. Worse still, they are systematically marginalized and underrepresented in governmental institutions and thus lacking in political empowerment (Zinsstag *et al.*, 2006). Most of the services required by the pastoral nomads can only be delivered under difficult circumstances. Pastoral nomads operate under relatively harsh climatic conditions, usually with low literacy level, conservative attitudes and mobile life. All these issues contribute to intense disease vulnerability among the pastoral nomads in Africa and elsewhere.

9.5 Meeting the Health Needs of African Pastoral Nomads: Some Core Principles

Having discussed some of the critical issues responsible for disease vulnerability among the pastoral nomads, it is important to draw lessons (or principles) from some best practices in meeting their healthcare needs (see Aliou, 1992; Schelling *et al.*, 2010; Montavon *et al.*, 2013; Ndiaye *et al.*, 2014; Shiekh and Kwaak, 2015). The polemic is that it is possible to meet the healthcare needs of the pastoral nomads if only one has strong political will (prioritization), a flexible approach and includes need principles and sustainable efforts (see Fig. 9.4).

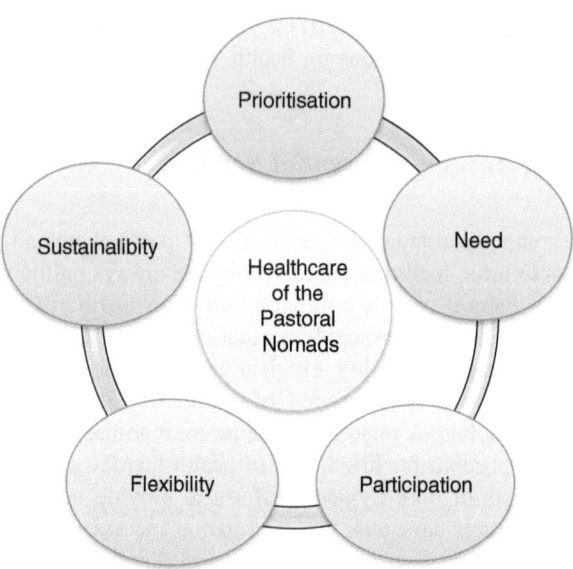

Fig. 9.4 Core principles in healthcare of pastoral nomads

9.5.1 Prioritization

The first major step in meeting the healthcare needs of the pastoral nomads is the understanding that the healthcare of any group is a priority. It is also important to understand that the pastoral nomads constitute a vulnerable and sociological group. There is a need for institutional commitment at all levels, both by state and non-state actors. One possibility would be to list pastoral nomads as a part of the vulnerable groups in healthcare delivery. There should be a concise effort to map pastoral communities and establish sustainable links with concerned agencies. The major flaw of the past is that the group has been marginalized and hardly recognized in international document as a distinct group with special needs, not only at state level but even by WHO (Zinsstag *et al.*, 2006). Priorization requires that resources be provided to pursue set health goals among the pastoral nomads. It involves policy recognition.

9.5.2 Need Principle

This principle involves a comprehensive assessment of the prerequisites for the pastoral nomads to attain the highest possible standard of health. By implication, it must address determinants of health, essential needs (e.g., food, water and sanitation) and actual healthcare (both for the pastoralists and animals). The need assessment cannot be complete without consideration of veterinary issues. This is not just necessitated due to cattle complex but also the One Health Approach. One of the major goals is to create access to healthcare (considering the various dimensions of access [see Sect. 1.3]). Universal coverage means that everyone is covered without any discrimination. While it may take painstaking efforts for some special groups, the overall health outcomes will benefit a lot if no group is excluded. Therefore, healthcare services should be extended to the pastoralist based on their needs.

9.5.3   Participation

It is also important that the pastoralists participate in every aspect of their healthcare. While there must be a strategic blueprint to cater for the healthcare needs of the group, consultation and involvement are key to promoting ownership and utilization of the services (see also Sect. 2.3.4). In fact, the group must be empowered with information and active involvement in the implementation of any program concerning them. Understanding the need and strategic approach to meet those needs are better derived from the perspective of those directly affected. This will also help to identify preferences, challenges and reservations. For instance, the success of polio vaccination among the pastoral nomads in Niger was partially attributed to the participation of the nomadic community leaders in the entire process (Ndiaye *et al.*, 2014).

9.5.4   Flexibility

It is important that healthcare is adaptable to the lifestyle of the pastoral nomads, if the pastoralists are to make efforts (when necessary and possible) to adjust to the healthcare designs. The bottom-line is that healthcare services should be flexible and considerate of the peculiar circumstances of the pastoral nomads. This is why Shiekh and Kwaak (2015) advocated for the development or use of nomadic health workers using the mobile clinic approach to reach the pastoral nomads. And Ndiaye *et al.* (2014) noted that the flexible services involving "vaccinators to adapt to circumstances and vaccinate when and where nomads were available or accessible, according to their seasonal movements and timing of life events" facilitate the extensive polio vaccination coverage of nomadic communities in Niger. It is also important to harmonize timing of activities between veterinarians and public health services (Schelling *et al.* 2010). Montavon *et al.* (2013) and Ndiaye *et al.* (2014) observed that the effective intersectoral collaboration between human and animal health services is vital for the overall success of health programs among the pastoral nomads.

9.5.5 Sustainability

It is also important that the design and inputs are sustainable. This should involve a simple technical know-how. This special need can be structured within an integrated primary healthcare, wherever the group exists. Aliou (1992) observed that independent mobile health units have proved to be ineffectual and excessively costly. Therefore, it is better to have a mobile unit within an already existing structure, such as a primary healthcare center but with wide radius of coverage to capture the pastoral nomads. Most times, the issue of sustainability has been the bane of healthcare programs in developing countries. There are a number of good best practices, which have been implemented in different regions but could not stand the test of time. There should be community structures, social networking and institutional support to ensure enduring strategic plans of action. Such sustainability will also guarantee that health programs become a normal part of pastoral life. This will invariably ensure better health outcomes, both in the short and long run.

References

Adriansen, H. K. (1997). *The development of nomadic pastoralism in Africa*. Copenhagen: Institute of Geography, University of Copenhagen.

Aliou, S. (1992). What health systems for nomadic population. *World Health Forum, 13*, 311–314.

Axweso, F. (2011). *Understanding pastoralists and their water, sanitation and hygiene needs. A discussion paper*. Dar es Salaam: WaterAid in Tanzania.

Blench, R. (2001). 'You can't go home again'. Pastoralism in the new millennium. https://www. odi.org/sites/odi.org.uk/files/odi-assets/publications-opinion-files/6329.pdf. Accessed 1 Jun 2016.

Chege, P. M., Kimiywe, J. O., Ndungu, Z. O. (2015). Influence of culture on dietary practices of children under five years among Maasai pastoralists in Kajiado, Kenya. *International Journal of Behavioral Nutrition and Physical Activity, 12*, 131. doi:10.1186/s12966-015-0284-3.

Desta, A. H. (2016). Pastoralism and the issue of zoonoses in Ethiopia. *Journal of Biology, Agriculture and Healthcare, 6*(7), 21–27.

Fratkin, E., Roth, E. A., Nathan, M. A. (2004). Pastoral sedentarization and its effects on children's diet, health, and growth among Rendille of Northern Kenya. *Human Ecology, 32*(5), 531–559.

IESS [International Encyclopedia of the Social Sciences] (2008). Pastoralism. http://www. encyclopedia.com/history/latin-america-and-caribbean/belizehistory/pastoral-systems. Accessed 15 May 2017.

Koocheki, A., & Gliessman, R. (2005). Pastoral nomadism: a sustainable system for grazing land management in arid areas. *Journal of Sustainable Agriculture, 25*(4), 113–131.

Loutan, L., & Lamotte, J. M. (1984). Seasonal variations in nutrition among a group of nomadic pastoralists in Niger. *The Lancet, 8383*(1), 945–947.

Mocellin, J., & Foggin, P. (2008). Health status and geographic mobility among semi-nomadic pastoralists in Mongolia. *Health & Place, 14*(2008), 228–242.

Montavon, A., Jean-Richard, V., Bechir, M., Daugla, D. M., Abdoulaye, M., Bongo Naré, R. N., et al. (2013). Health of mobile pastoralists in the Sahel—assessment of 15 years of research and development. *Tropical Medicine and International Health, 18*(9), 1044–1052.

Moritz, M., Ewing, D., Garabed, R. B. (2013). On not knowing zoonotic diseases: pastoralists' ethnoveterinary knowledge in the far north region of Cameroon. *Human Organization, 72*(1), 1–11.

Muhammad-Baba, T. A., & Amzat, J. (2012). Pastoralism, nomadism and transhumance: an explanation of the socio-economic organization of Fulani/Ful'be of northern Nigeria. In A. S. Jegede, A. O. Olutayo, O. Omololu & B. E. Owumi (Eds.), *Peoples and cultures of Nigeria* (pp. 78–96). Ibadan: Department of Sociology, University of Ibadan.

Ndiaye, S. M., Ahmed, M. A., Denson, M., Craig, A. S., Kretsinger, K., Cherif, B., et al. (2014). Polio outbreak among nomads in Chad: outbreak response and lessons learned. *The Journal of Infectious Diseases*, *210*(S1), S74–S84. doi:10.1093/infdis/jit564.

Oba, G., & Lusigi, W. J. (1987). An overview of drought strategies and land use in African pastoral systems. Paper 23a. https://www.odi.org/sites/odi.org.uk/files/odi-assets/publications-opinion-files/5285.pdf Accessed 1 Jun 2016.

Okeibuinor, J. C., Onyeneho, N. J., Nwaorgu, O. C., I'Aronu, N., Okoye, I., Iremeka, F. U., et al. (2013). Prospects of using community directed intervention strategy in delivering health services among Fulani Nomads in Enugu State, Nigeria. *International Journal for Equity in Health*, *12*, 24.

Randall, S. (2010). Nomads, refugees and repatriates: histories of mobility and health outcomes in northern Mali. *Society, Biology and Human Affairs*, *75*(2), 1–26.

Randall, S. (2015). Where have all the nomads gone? Fifty years of statistical and demographic invisibilities of African mobile pastoralists. *Pastoralism: Research, Policy and Practice*, *5*, 22. doi:10.1186/s13570-015-0042-9.

Rota, A., & Sperandini, S. (2009). Livestock and pastoralists. Livestcok Thematic Paper. https://www.ifad.org/documents/10180/0fbe4134-4354-4d08-bf09-e1a6dbee3691. Accessed 30 May 2016.

Salzman, P. C. (2004). *Pastoralists: equality, hierarchy, and the state*. Oxford: Westview Press.

Schelling, E. (2002). Human and animal health in nomadic pastoralist communities of Chad: zoonoses, morbidity and health services. PhD Dissertation Submitted to University of Basel, Basel, Switzerland.

Schelling, E., Béchir, M., Daugla, D. M., Bonfoh, B., Tableb, M. O., Zinsstag, J., et al. (2010). Health research among highly mobile pastoralist communities of Chad. *Society, Biology & Human Affairs*, *75*, 93–113.

Sheik-Mohamed, A., & Velema, J. P. (1999). Where healthcare has no access: the nomadic populations of sub-Saharan Africa. *Tropical Medicine and International Health*, *4*(10), 695–707.

Shiekh, B., & Kwaak, A. (2015). Factors influencing the utilization of maternal health care services by nomads in Sudan. *Pastoralism: Research, Policy and Practice*, *5*, 23. doi:10.1186/s13570-015-0041-x.

Smith, A. B. (1992a). *Pastoralism in Africa: origins and development ecology*. London, UK: Hurst and Co Publishers.

Smith, A. B. (1992b). Origins and spread of pastoralism in Africa. *Annual Review of Anthropology*, *21*, 125–141.

Smith, A. B. (2005). Origins and spread of African pastoralism. *History Compass*, *4*(1), 1–7.

Swift, J., Toulmin C., Chatting S. (1990). Providing services for nomadic people—a review of the literature and annotated bibliography. In UNICEF staff working papers number 8, UNICEF, New York.

Taylor, L. H., Latham, S. M., Woolhouse, M. E. (2001). Risk factors for disease emergence. *Philosophical Transactions: Biological Science, Royal Society of London*, *356*(1411), 983–989.

Wurzinger, M., Ndumu, D., Okeyo, A. M., Sölkner, J. (2011). Lifestyle and herding practices of Bahima pastoralists in Uganda. *African Journal of Agricultural Research*, *3*(8), 542–548.

Zinsstag, J., Taleb, M. O., Craig, P. S. (2006). Editorial: health of nomadic pastoralists: new approaches towards equity effectiveness. *Tropical Medicine and International Health*, *11*(5), 565–568.

Chapter 10
Healthcare Emergencies in Africa: The Case of Ebola in Nigeria

10.1 Introduction

Since the first outbreak of Ebola Virus Disease (EVD) in 1976 in Congo (DR) and Sudan (now South Sudan), it has claimed hundreds of lives and remains one of the most dreadful viral infections in human history (WHO, 1978). At different points in time (before 2014), EVD outbreaks had previously occurred in Congo (DR); Sudan (the region is now a part of South Sudan), Uganda, Gabon, Cote d'Ivoire and South Africa. Guinea, Liberia, Sierra Leone and Nigeria joined the list of countries with Ebola outbreaks in 2014. Ebola is highly contagious through minimal contact with any sufferer and has the potential to develop into a pandemic. EVD outbreaks have a case fatality rate of up to 90% (WHO, 2014a). In 2014, the outbreak occurred for the first time in four countries simultaneously, in addition to imported cases recorded in the USA, Spain and Saudi Arabia. At that point the outbreak was considered a global public health emergency (WHO, 2014b). It has been observed that, as a result of increased international travel and trade, local outbreaks of infectious diseases (like EVD) often acquire international importance (Grein *et al.*, 2000). The 2014/2015 Ebola outbreak started in March (2014) in Guinea, later spread to Sierra Leone and then to Liberia. Nigeria joined the list when it recorded an imported case on July 20, 2014.

The 2014–2015 outbreaks were the worst in history, affecting several countries even beyond Africa. The worst hit countries were Guinea, Liberia and Sierra Leone, accounting for 28,616 confirmed cases with 11,310 deaths (WHO, 2016). The Ebola situation in the worst hit countries lasted up into 2016; they were declared Ebola-free in June 2016. In the beginning of the crisis, it was a situation of inadequate capacity and weak political will to manage the transmission of the virus. With the global emergency declared, there were numerous supportive measures, which helped to eventually end of the crisis. But within

J. Amzat, O. Razum, *Towards a Sociology of Health Discourse in Africa*, DOI 10.1007/978-3-319-61672-8_10 the same time frame, Nigeria was able to manage its EVD outbreak within a short period. The essence of this chapter is not to focus on the history of horrors and crises generated by Ebola in West Africa, but to focus on the Nigerian example of how the disease was successfully managed, and draw lessons for future pandemics.

Following this background, the chapter examines the politics and ethics of EVD in Nigeria from the date of contact with a carrier from Liberia. The chapter also examines some public reactions, especially associated-panic with the outbreak of the virus. The defining indicators of this incubation period, like in other outbreaks, involved the risk of EVD—its perception; communication (dissemination of information to the public); management (containment strategies, healthcare frontline and government response [e.g., mobilization of resources]); and community mobilization (local understanding, social referrals, contact tracing and risk avoidance)—which should serve as cardinal points in the fight against the virus (see Smith, 2006).

10.2 Ebola in Nigeria

On July 20, Mr. Patrick Sawyer, a Liberian-American (naturalized American who was also an official in the Liberian government) flew into Nigeria from Liberia. He became severely ill upon arrival (unknowingly at the initial stage), however, Ebola was not suspected. Several people, especially healthcare givers freely interacted with Mr. Sawyer without any protective medical kits that could potentially protect against a dreadful disease like Ebola. After 2 days, Ebola was suspected. This was the beginning of the clamor that Ebola was in Lagos, Nigeria. This signifies that the first case was an imported case. Mr. Sawyer died 3 days later. Nigeria was forced to face the reality that EVD has been imported and that all of Mr. Sawyer's primary contacts were at risk of contracting the disease. This was the beginning of the politics, ethical concerns, and general public panic.

Following the aforementioned incidence, the primary concern of the government was monitoring the primary contacts of the index case, given the fact that the incubation period of EVD is 2–21 days. By implication, the primary contacts could only be considered free of EVD if there was no medical indication after 21 days. In the case of Nigeria, the period started from the date of arrival of Mr. Sawyer, July 20–August 9, 2014. Cases detected were difficult to manage, as the patients required intensive supportive care and there was no licensed/registered treatment or vaccine for EVD (WHO, 2014a). A similar situation occurred in Uganda from October 8, 2000–January 16, 2001 (Okware et al., 2002). It also required following up patients and contacts for 21 days. During the period, a total of 425 cases with 224 deaths were reported; nearly 5000 contacts were followed up for 21 days (Okware et al., 2002). Uganda was finally certified Ebola free on February 27, 2001, which was 42 days after the last case was reported.

10.2.1 The Growing Number of Victims

In general, apart from family members of the sufferers (intra-familial spread) (see Baron, Mccormick, & Zubeir, 1983), the next set of people most at risk of EVD are healthcare workers (Khan *et al.*, 1999). For instance, during the outbreak in DR Congo (DR) in 1995, 80 cases (25%) occurred among healthcare workers (Khan *et al.*, 1999). In the case of Liberia, the senior physician, Samuel Brisbane, on the frontline of Ebola treatment contracted the virus and died. Similarly, an American doctor, Kent Brantly, and an Ebola doctor in Sierra Leone, Sheik Umar, were infected (Yan & Levs, 2014). In Nigeria as well, the physician, Stella Adadevoh, who treated Mr. Sawyer became symptomatic, hence she was the first Nigerian case of Ebola declared. The second death was also one of the nurses who cared for the American-Liberian. Another nurse who came into contact with Mr. Sawyer tested positive and was quarantined, while her husband was kept under surveillance. Gradually, Nigeria faced a growing number of victims. It was apparent that the health workers had been unaware of the Ebola status of Mr. Sawyer, therefore, adequate preventive and protective measures were not followed. Following the revelation that the American-Liberian (the index case) died of Ebola, the government went swiftly into action by monitoring all those who had had direct contact with the index case. Within a week, the Lagos state government announced that over 50 people were being monitored.

As expected, the virus proved to be highly infectious; within 21 days, there were 10 confirmed cases. Many of the confirmed cases were quarantined and an isolated unit was established at the Mainland Hospital in Lagos. While the number of cases was still few at this stage, the effectiveness of a control strategy depends on the adherence to infection control guidelines, surveillance strategies and public participation. This was not the right time to contemplate how to avoid an Ebola explosion in Nigeria. Given the Nigerian circumstances (doctors' strike, open borders, public panic and communal orientation), proactive measures should have started long before the arrival of Mr. Sawyer in Nigeria. The arrival could have been prevented in the first instance if, considering his country of origin, his condition would have been treated immediately as a suspected case of EVD.

As of early August 2014, the case fatality in Nigeria stood at 28.6%. The victims could still be hopeful in the light of this scientific fact, but considering the doctors' strike and the fact that this was the first Ebola crisis in Nigeria, there was a perceived pessimism regarding the survival rate. As of August 8, there were 139 persons under close monitoring; they included those who had had contact with the index case and secondary contacts. The figure would have been higher had some contacts not "escaped" monitoring by deliberately moving to other States of the federation. One of the "escapees," a nurse who was a primary contact with the late Mr. Sawyer, moved to another State (Enugu State, about 560 km away from Lagos). Before being quarantined again, the nurse had contact with 21 more people in Enugu. It was because of this development that the then Minister of Health expressed great worry that other States (apart from Lagos) might also be at risk of EVD. This accounted for more concern, both in nearby States and in neighboring countries, especially Ghana, Togo and Benin Republic.

10.2.2   Beyond the First 21 Days

The proactive efforts continued, but with some challenges. Additional measures were put in place to further contain the spread of EVD. Public enlightenment and lectures were intensified among various groups: market women, auto mechanics, traders, artisans, prison inmates, students, health workers, etc. More isolation centers were established across the country, but resistance was recorded in some communities. There were protests in Kakuri (Kaduna State) and Emuoha (Rivers State) against situating an isolation center in their communities. Many community members believed such centers could increase their risk, and hence vulnerability to EVD infection.

The number of EVD cases remained stable and treatment was yielding some positive results, especially within the first 37 days. As of the 38th day, (August 26, 2014), all reported cases had root in the index case, resulting in 5 deaths (apart from the index case) and 7 treated and discharged; 129 people completed the incubation period without any symptoms; and 128 people remained under surveillance. The efforts of the government were applauded both locally and internationally. As for those individuals who had evaded quarantine or monitoring: the nurse who was returned to quarantine from Enugu on August 28 and a doctor who had been treating one of the (ECOWAS) diplomats (who had had contact with the Lagos index case and had evaded quarantine to another city [Port Harcourt, about 612 km from Lagos]) both died of EVD (Ibeh, 2014). The Port Harcourt physician invariably became that city's EVD index case. He put many other individuals at risk: when they visited his home for a christening ceremony; when he continued to treat patients at his private hospital; when he was treated by other physicians when he became symptomatic; when, for a few days after his death, many people paid condolence visits to his home; and when the body was deposited in a hospital morgue. It was on August 27 that the case was confirmed (WHO, 2014c). The widow of the Port Harcourt index case (also a physician) became symptomatic; hence, two additional reported cases. This put the number of additional people who had contact with the diplomat and the deceased doctor under surveillance to nearly 200.

The Port Harcourt scenario was a case of serial denial. Critically, the escapee put several others in danger by seeking private treatment without the knowledge of the health authorities. The deceased doctor did not adhere to the repeated public health warnings. This led to renewed efforts of contact tracing and public apprehension at a time the when country was close to declaring zero cases of EVD. Invariably, the Nigeria EVD status had to be updated, as shown in Table 10.1.

Table 10.1 Ebola in Nigeria: final data

Deaths	8
Total reported cases	20
Released from surveillance	Over 300
No. of affected states	3 (Lagos, Enugu and Rivers)

10.3   The Politics of Ebola: Some Governmental Responses/Countermeasures

As noted earlier, the first priority of the government was to monitor those who had had contact with the index case for 21 days (the incubation period of the virus). Within this period, nine confirmed cases, apart from the index case, were established, with one dead. Those confirmed cases, must also have had contact with others in the society, putting even more people at risk for EVD. As a consequence, on August 7, the Federal Government of Nigeria (FGN) declared a National Emergency on Ebola. The Nigerian President also earmarked 1.9b Naira (around $11m) for containment strategies following an approved Special Intervention Plan (SIP) to further strengthen on-going steps to contain the virus. The President charged the Federal Ministry of Health to work in collaboration with the State Ministries of Health, the National Centre for Disease Control (NCDC), the National Emergency Management Agency (NEMA) and other relevant agencies to implement containment strategies in line with international protocols and best practices in order to curb the threat of EVD in Nigeria. The SIP includes active Ebola surveillance through contact tracing, temperature examination at international airports for outbound and inbound passengers, establishment of isolation centers, procurement of required equipment and deployment of staff. A similar emergency was declared in Liberia, where schools and borders were closed and $18m earmarked to facilitate containment strategies.

The state government of Lagos reacted sharply, knowing that EVD is a dire health emergency. There was a press conference involving neighboring states. This prompted some States of the federation to set up isolation centers. The Governor of Lagos donated 268m Naira to 134 schools for personal hygiene as part of the fight against Ebola.

As at August 8, 2014, WHO had reported that 961 people had died from Ebola in West Africa, 2 of them in Nigeria. The total number of cases was 1779—despite the fact that more cases were still evolving through investigation, this was already the highest number of confirmed cases in the history of EVD outbreaks. Consequently, on August 8, WHO declared the Ebola outbreak in West Africa a Public Health Emergency of International Concern (PHEIC) and noted that "the possible consequences of further international spread are particularly serious in view of the virulence of the virus, the intensive community and health facility transmission patterns, and the weak health systems in the currently affected and most at-risk countries." (WHO, 2014b). One of the vital recommendations of WHO (2014b) was that there should be a large-scale and sustained effort to fully engage the community to play a key role in case identification, contact tracing and risk education. In fact, response to the EVD outbreak in the Congo (DR) in 1995 involved house-to-house searches, which helped in rapid identification of cases (Khan et al. 1995).

While a state of emergency was declared on EVD in Nigeria, the doctors' strike was still on-going. This provided a basis of appeal to the striking doctors to suspend strike action to assist in containing the viral disease. On the contrary, the doctors insisted on their demands (including upgrading of hospital facilities and welfare package), hence the strike continued. Therefore, calls for volunteers went out, with an offer to give those who came forward life insurance.

The USA also has two imported cases from Liberia who were airlifted to the USA for better treatment. The cases were quarantined and treated at Emory University Hospital. The main drug, the experimental Ebola Serum (unapproved) called ZMapp, was used. When the patients showed some signs of improvement, the affected West African countries, including Nigeria, were optimistic that the USA would make the experimental drug available. Nigeria, through the Minister of Health, made a request for the experimental drug, which, for several reasons, was turned down by the USA. Although there were still pertinent ethical questions regarding the use of the drug, many health experts advocated for the experimental drugs to be provided to the affected African countries. However, the USA argued that, as they were only treating two patients at the time, in the event of serious adverse events, the damage would be very minimal in terms of causalities or fatalities (and related unexpected consequences). If such a drug was widely used in regions with thousands of cases, the situation could be worse. There was still the need to assess the drugs in terms of unexpected events, dosage, and adverse events. More importantly, the supply was still not adequate to meet the demands of the Ebola-affected countries. The sick, who are regarded as vulnerable, were less concerned about possible adverse events since, in the absence any effective treatment, they are likely to die. Most lay people in the affected countries still could not comprehend why such ethical concerns were prioritized in the face of Ebola death toll.

One critical concern in the Nigerian case was about the hundreds of open and unmanned borders across all the regions of Nigeria. Perhaps, the FGN had less apprehension about those borders because the first case was actually imported by air. However, along these lines, the FGN did suspend Air Gambia from flying into Nigeria, since it was the main airline flying passengers from Liberia, Sierra Leone and Guinea into Nigeria (Adekola, 2014). This was an effort to stop additional imported case. As the number of victims grew, so did the possibility that other countries would also suspend receiving flights from Nigeria. This would have placed a great burden on Nigeria, since it has a huge population flying daily into several countries of the world. Such suspension of flights might have been tantamount to "socioeconomic sanction" and accrued tremendous burden on the nation's economy. Luckily, such a ban was never promulgated.

The mainstay of the Nigeria's success was a rapid, national, multisectoral response. It was the same scenario in Uganda, which also showed a "strong national multisectoral mobilization, which provided essential coordination and mobilized resources" (Okware et al. 2002). In Nigeria, news centers were designated and, most importantly, a health emergency was declared. Although this was the first time Nigeria had faced an Ebola crisis, even within the incubation period, the containment strategies were effective and sustained.

10.4   Public Panic and the Search for a Local Remedy

Historically, infectious diseases have often cause public panic and social distress (such was the case of HIV, SARS, EVD, Avian Influenza, Cholera, Lassa Fever and Meningitis). The peculiarities of infectious disease often make the entire world to be greatly apprehensive. An occurrence in one country could easily transmit to another country if not effectively managed and safeguarded. Such diseases often attract major news headlines across the world, and thus become a global issue. And while a number of countries might be setting up control or treatment measures, others will be immersed in protective frameworks. The apprehension often moves from the political to the social level (especially at the level of the individual), following perceived possibility of transmissions.

Smith *et al.* (2004:2) assert that "[T]he individual fear and community panic associated with infectious diseases often leads to rapid, emotionally driven decision making about public health policies needed to protect the community that may be in conflict with current bioethical principles regarding the care of individual patients." In Africa, reactions are also traditionally driven, often leading to unscientific or crude responses to the threat. It is often possible for "uncommon scenarios" to be attributed to supernatural and mystical causes (Amzat & Razum, 2014). Controlling misconceptions and reinforcing scientifically valid evidence should be a major priority of both the media and the government (Okware *et al.*, 2002). It is important for the media to shift from "alarming" to reassuring and educative coverage (see Ungar, 1998). This was why, during the recent Ebola outbreak, the Nigerian government set up a media center led by the Minister of Health to report the state of the outbreak on a daily basis. Part of the mandate of the media center was also to address publicly circulated information about the virus and to debunk Ebola myths. This is also a kind of rumor surveillance, which is aimed at decreasing "the potential for misinformation and misunderstanding and to inform the public and health officials about disease outbreaks, facilitate a rapid response, and promote public health preparedness" (Samaan *et al.*, 2005, p. 463).

The communicability of EVD also generated panic that affected patterns of interaction in the society. This amplified public panic and led to various declarations of emergencies in Nigeria (both the Federal and State governments) and other affected countries (Guinea, Liberia and Sierra Leone). People began to query patterns of normal intimacy and general interactions. For instance, hugging, handshakes and general body contact were only undertaken with cautions. This pattern was seen not only in Lagos, where there were confirmed cases, but across several nations. While some will argue that the threshold of infection was still low to affect pattern of interaction, perhaps, it is medically recommended to be preventive irrespective of the level of perceived risk. Travel advisories were issued to countries with prolonged incidence. Many countries advised their citizen to be cautious about traveling to affected countries, while flight from those countries were also suspended.

Public panic was a reflection of the low rate of survival—only about 1–40% would survive. Survival during disease outbreaks also depends on the healthcare system. The rate of survival also varies from individual to individual. In the Nigerian case, the symptomatic physician outlives the second person (a nurse), who died shortly after presenting with symptoms. This acuity or acuteness of EVD precipitates rapid actions among the public and generated a lot of experimentation with local remedies. More importantly, it could also lead to mistrust of the modern healthcare system. While most people are aware that survival rate is low, in the face of Nigeria doctors' strike, it could be lower as there might not be adequate care especially if the number of cases increases. In fact, Mr. Sawyer was treated in a private hospital since the doctors working in public hospital were on strike.

The level of public panic greatly depends on the level of awareness and knowledge. The general ignorance about causes, modes of transmission, levels of vulnerability, self-efficacy, and outcomes often engender "fear of the unknown, and possible over-reaction by public health officials in the use of isolation and quarantine" (Smith et al., 2004:4). The ignorance often leads to misconceptions. For instance, many in Nigeria erroneously claimed that Ebola is airborne; in Sierra Leone, many relatives aggressively requested for the release of the corpse of their relatives in order to perform some burial rites, not understanding that a corpse can still spread the disease. Apart from this, there is often the problem of self-efficacy—that is ability to self-manage and implement effective action. In the context of Ebola, avoiding social contacts with people suspected of being infected can be problematic, especially when they are still asymptomatic. Contacting EVD is generally regarded as a death sentence because of the unavailability of a known cure at the moment, and the fear of isolation/quarantine could prevent a number of people from reporting their status, suspicion or risk. In the first 21 days in Nigeria (as previously observed), many secondary contacts "escaped" monitoring, thereby posing great concern/risk to the general public.

With the news of the outbreak of Ebola in Nigeria, the first reaction of many was a conspiracy theory. The critical issues were: did Mr. Sawyer escape quarantine in Liberia? Why did the Liberian government allow him to travel "knowing" that he was at risk as a secondary contact following the burial of his sister who died of EVD? Why did Mr. Sawyer deny any possibility of risk of Ebola directing the attention to a suspected case of malaria? While Mr. Sawyer was not alive to defend the circumstances surrounding his travel to Nigeria, he was being persecuted. The reason for the persecution was obvious within the incubation period of the EVD. In fact Nigerian President described him as a "crazy" man (Odunsi, 2014). The government was also concerned about tracing those who had contacts with the dead American-Liberian. The public was almost overwhelmed with anxiety. Even those who are thousand kilometers away from Lagos were in panic about the report of EVD, because Lagos is characterized with massive inflow and outflow of people. The realization was that detection of EVD in Lagos could spell a common destiny for all of Nigeria unless effective measures of containment were sustained. In general, the public reaction was positive in stopping the spread of Ebola.

Another dimension of the public fear emanates from the particular features of EVD. WHO (2014a) observed that EVD is a severe acute viral illness often characterized by the sudden onset of fever, intense weakness, muscle pain and headache. But the disease has symptom complex—it manifests like many common diseases (including malaria). Fever (for instance) is a major symptomatic manifestation of malaria. With the high prevalence of malaria in West Africa, every occurrence of high fever might engender unwarranted nervousness. This could also lead to a number of misdiagnoses, while those with fever might tend to conceal it for fear of being quarantined or mistaken for EVD.

Regarding the search for cure, it has been previously mentioned that there could be traditionally- or misconception-driven prescriptions. That was the case in Nigeria after the first case was recorded. Just like the news of EVD, the "news" spread quickly that the beverage Gracina Kola (often called bitter kola in Nigeria) could cure Ebola. The assertion was credited to a professor of pharmacology in Nigeria, Maurice Iwu, based on inconclusive research in 1999 showing in-vitro that Gracina Kola could halt the growth and reproduction of the virus. Without any further clarification from Iwu, the "prescription" was circulated across every available means of communication, especially through the social media (Facebook, BBM, Twitter, WhatsApp, Viber, etc). This triggered a mass demand for Gracina Kola, and consequently, its price tripled. It also led to a scarcity of Gracina Kola across Nigeria within 24 hours. The FGN and scientific community later debunked the claim about the potency of Gracina Kola against EVD. The announcement was a mark of disappointment for many looking towards Gracina Kola as a probable cure against EVD.

A few days after the refutation of the potency of Gracina Kola, there was another announcement that salt-water solution could protect against EVD. The announcement was purportedly made by one of the traditional rulers in Nigeria (Ogala, Ibeh, & Audu, 2014). The prescription was received with great enthusiasm, as Nigerians exchanged telephone calls advising one another to drink and bathe with salt-water solution (Ogala *et al.*, 2014). A text quickly spread asserting that, "to prevent Ebola sickness, use hot salt water to bathe before 4am." Another text added that people should recite some protective verses from the bible or Quran into the salt water. Many Nigerians had to wake up from sleep to perform the ritual of drinking and bathing with salt water. The "enthusiasm" was short-lived, as FGN issued a statement that salt-water has no potent ingredient against EVD.

Rumor surveillance was a major task during the outbreak. There were daily press briefings to clarify the situations and provide useful information for the general public on preventive measures. The rumors were promptly debunked.

10.5 Ethical Concerns Relating to Ebola Outbreak in Nigeria

Health emergencies, such as the outbreaks of SARS and EVD require prompt actions, which are often fraught with moral perplexities. It is in this light that Ovadia, Gazit, Silner, and Kagan (2005) averred that decision-making in a time of emergency and outbreak is associated with a high potential of ethical dilemmas. Smith *et al.* (2004, 2006) also noted that ethical issues arise in infectious diseases because of their powerful ability to generate panic in populations. The EVD outbreak in 2014 generated concerns at the global level, and prompted WHO to declare an international health emergency. While WHO did not recommend a closing of borders, it warned that every traveler should be screened (WHO, 2014b). Mandatory screening at airports and borders negate the principle of autonomy and privacy. On any suspicion of high fever, a traveler might be subjected to further screening, denied right of movement at that moment, and if there is any other positive indication, the traveler might be quarantined.

While the persons with positive EVD status and their family members might object to such isolation, the medical protocol in the management of EVD and related disease is sacrosanct. This is necessary because EVD can be passed from one individual to another through various forms of contact. As Smith *et al.* (2004) observed the mode of transmission of infectious diseases (such as EVD and SARS) also raises questions of responsibility, since the infected individual poses a risk to others in the society. Self-referral and conformity with medical protocol of isolation are encouraged as a sign of responsibility and protection of significant others and others in the society. But in the case of Nigeria (as earlier observed), many suspected persons fled monitoring, and could have been responsible had the disease spread beyond only the affected State and scope of current surveillance of primary context with the index case.

Regarding the potential success of treatment with ZMapp in the USA, there are still some pressing questions beyond what was earlier noted. Before any American became infected, there was no mention of any "available" and promising experimental drug in the USA. Perhaps, the world might not be aware of any promising drugs if no American was infected. Sometimes, an act of omission could constitute a vital breach of ethics and humanitarian gesture. This should prompt the WHO to revisit the ethics of drug distribution in the face of highly infectious and deadly diseases like EVD and SARS.

In addition, regarding the use of experimental drugs in Nigeria, Clement Adebamowo, the Chairman, National Health Research Ethics Committee of Nigeria (NHRECN) issued a national policy statement reiterating the ethical permissibility of the use of innovative or non-validated medical treatment designed solely for the benefits of the patient during EVD emergency without any application or prior approval by NHRECN (Adebamowo, 2014). In order to facilitate the prompt international response to the global EVD emergency, the NHRECN also waived the requirement that the establishment of a Material Transfer Agreement (MTA) should precede international shipment of biological samples out of Nigeria (Adebamowo, 2014). This waiver would enable the shipment of samples for further laboratory tests.

Apart from ethical issues at the national level, there are social consequences of epidemics. The EVD (like most infectious diseases) exacts significant impact on pattern of social interaction. In the case of EVD, handshakes and other forms of casual physical contact were discouraged. The Ebola emergency also forced the Catholic Church to suspend the rite or sign of peace during mass (which involve handshaking among congregants) (Ibekwe, 2014). Due to the warning that fruit bats are natural hosts of Ebola virus and that other forest animals were under suspicion, consumption of animals from hunting was highly discouraged. Consequently, the household economy of those who specialize in trading such animals was adversely affected. Cremation and mass burial in cemeteries far away from populated areas meant that families were forced to go against traditional arrangements and forego rites (Okware *et al.* 2002). As the government might take possession of the body and bury it according to the health emergency protocol, the family might not even be allowed to see the body of the deceased (see Gostin, Lucey, & Phelan, 2014).

Another critical ethical concern is whether the refusal of the striking doctors to call off the strike should be considered as a neglect of duty (of care). The strike began approximately 2 weeks before the first case of EVD in Nigeria. The declaration of the national emergency should depend greatly on the health workers especially physicians. Iserson *et al.* (2008) rightly observed that most public health emergency plans often rely on physicians, nurses, emergency department support staff, and out-of-hospital personnel to maintain the healthcare system's front line. Perhaps, if some of them return as volunteers despite the strike, this could be humanitarian enough in conformity with some level of duty of care. A nurse on leave from Emory University Hospital exhibited altruistic practice and duty of care by returning to work to care for the American Ebola victims brought from Liberia. It could be argued that moral responsibility, duty of care and national interest override the right of healthcare workers to strike.

From the foregoing, there is no doubt that the outbreak of EVD (like other infectious diseases) raised ethical concerns; Fear of infection offers numerous opportunities to defy bioethical principles such as autonomy, beneficence, non-maleficence, privacy, and other human rights-based considerations (e.g., right to movement and association). In the face of EVD, the needs and rights of populations and certain individuals might be breached as a result of disease screening and quarantine (Smith *et al.*, 2004, p. 2). In the case of health emergencies, individuals have a societal obligation to cooperate with health and other instituted authorities in crisis management. It took the Liberian government some military involvement to curtail the movements of people in some affected quarters. In Nigeria, evading monitoring by some individuals was against public health interest and highly unethical. It is in this light that Calain, Fiore, Poncin, and Hurst (2009:7) submitted that EVD outbreak "can be seen as a paradigm for ethical issues posed by epidemic emergencies, through the convergence of such themes as: isolation and quarantine, privacy and confidentiality and the interpretation of ethical norms across different ethnocultural settings" (Calain *et al.*, 2009, p. 7), including the use of experimental drugs, contact tracing and monitoring and compulsory disease screening.

10.6 Conclusion

Nigeria was eventually declared Ebola-free on October 19, 2014. Overall, the Nigerian experience was a success story with some important lessons. As earlier observed, Nigeria was not prepared for the prevention of such an emergency. When it was clear that some West African countries were already inflicted with the crisis,

Nigeria should have taken some precautionary measures, such as airport screening of persons from those countries. Perhaps the index case could have been stopped and isolated at the airport. Whether in the throes of a crisis or not, precautionary preparedness is always recommended; the instituted capacity to manage Ebola should not be completely dismantled. The swift response and multisectoral mobilization, including information dissemination, were the real magic used to end the Ebola crisis in Nigeria.

References

Adebamowo, C. (2014). Statement on the use of innovative or non-validated medical treatment in Nigeria. A statement issued on August 9, 2014, by the Chair, National Health Research Ethics Committee, Nigeria During National Emergency on Ebola.

Adekola, S. (2014). Why NCAA Suspended Air Gambia from Nigeria. http://www.tribune.com. ng/news/news-headlines/item/12987-why-ncaa-suspended-air-gambia-from-nigeria. Accessed 12 Aug 2014.

Amzat, J., & Razum, O. (2014). *Medical sociology in Africa*. Switzerland: Springer International Publishing.

Baron, R. C., Mccormick, J. B., Zubeir, O. A. (1983). Ebola virus disease in southern Sudan: hospital dissemination and intrafamilial spread. *Bulletin of the World Health Organization, 61*(6), 997–1003.

Calain, P., Fiore, N., Poncin, M., Hurst, S. A. (2009). Research ethics and international epidemic response: the case of Ebola and Marburg hemorrhagic fevers. *Public Health Ethics, 2*(1), 7–29. doi:10.1093/phe/phn037.

Gostin, L. O., Lucey, D., Phelan, A. (2014). The Ebola epidemic: a global health emergency. *JAMA*, E1-E2. doi:10.1001/jama.2014.11176.

Grein, T. W., Kamara, K. O., Rodier, G., Plant, A. J., Bovier, P., Ryan, M. J., et al. (2000). Rumors of disease in the global village: outbreak verification. *Emerging Infectious Diseases, 6*(2), 98–102.

Ibeh, N. (2014). Diplomat, who took Ebola to Rivers, an ECOWAS staff—See more at: https://www.premiumtimesng.com/featured-news/167472-diplomat-who-took-ebola-to-rivers-an-ecowas-staff.html#sthash.3x4W2NQ5.dpuf. Accessed 29 Aug 2014.

Ibekwe, N. (2014). Ebola: Catholic Church suspends 'sign of peace' ritual during Mass. https://www.premiumtimesng.com/news/top-news/166480-ebola-catholic-church-suspends-sign-of-peace-ritual-during-mass.html#sthash.X8uWcF1Y.dpbs. Accessed 11 Aug 2014.

Iserson, K. V., Heine, C. E., Larkin, G. L., Moskop, J. C., Baruch, J., Aswegan, A. L. (2008). Fight or flight: the ethics of emergency physician disaster response. *Annals of Emergency Medicine, 51*, 345–353.

Khan, A. S., Tshioko, F. K., Heymann, D. L., Le Guenno, B., Nabeth, P., Kerstiëns, B., et al. (1999). The reemergence of Ebola hemorrhagic fever, Democratic Republic of the Congo, 1995. *Journal of Infectious Diseases, 179*(Suppl 1), S76–S86. doi:10.1086/514306.

Odunsi, W. (2014). Ebola: Sawyer's trip to Nigeria infuriates Jonathan, calls him a 'crazy man.' http://dailypost.ng/2014/08/11/ebola-sawyers-trip-nigeria-infuriates-jonathan-calls-crazy-man/. Accessed 12 Aug 2014.

Ogala, E., Ibeh, E., Audu, O. (2014). Ebola sparks panic across Nigeria as citizens scramble for salt-water bath "remedy". *Premium Times*, https://www.premiumtimesng.com/?p=166257?p=166257#sthash.PuhcwRNx.dpbs. Accessed 9 Aug 2014.

Okware, S. I., Omaswa, F. G., Opio, Z., Lutwama, A., Kamugisha, J. J., Rwaguma, J., et al. (2002). An outbreak of Ebola in Uganda. *Tropical Medicine and International Health, 7*(12), 1068–1075.

Ovadia, K. L., Gazit, I., Silner, D., Kagan, I. (2005). Better late than never: a re-examination of ethical dilemmas in coping with severe acute respiratory syndrome. *Journal of Hospital Infection*, *61*, 75–79.

Samaan, G., Patel, M., Olowokure, B., Roces, M. C., Oshitani, H., the World Health Organization Outbreak Response Team (2005). Rumor surveillance and avian influenza H5N1. *Emerging Infectious Diseases*, *11*(3), 463–466.

Smith, C. B., Battin, M. P., Jacobson, J. A., Francis, L. P., Botkin, J. R., Asplund, E. P., et al. (2004). Are there characteristics of infectious diseases that raise special ethical issues? *Developing World Bioethics*, *4*(1), 1–16.

Smith, R. D. (2006). Responding to global infectious disease outbreaks: lessons from SARS on the role of risk perception, communication and management. *Social Science & Medicine*, *63*, 3113–3123.

Ungar, S. (1998). Hot crises and media reassurance: a comparison of emerging diseases and Ebola Zaire. *The British Journal of Sociology*, *49*(1), 36–56.

WHO [World Health Organization] (1978). Ebola haemorrhagic fever in Zaire, 1976. Report of an International Convention. *Bulletin of the World Health Organization*, *56*(2), 271–293.

WHO [World Health Organization] (2014a). Ebola Virus Disease. http://www.who.int/mediacentre/factsheets/fs103/en/. Accessed 9 Aug 2014.

WHO [World Health Organization] (2014b).WHO Statement on the meeting of the international health regulations emergency committee cegarding the 2014 Ebola outbreak in West Africa. http://www.who.int/mediacentre/news/statements/2014/ebola-20140808/en/. Accessed 10 Aug 2014.

WHO [World Health Organization] (2014c). Ebola situation in Port Harcourt, Nigeria. http://who.int/mediacentre/news/ebola/3-september-2014/en/. Accessed 5 Sep 2014.

WHO [World Health Organization] (2016). Situation report: Ebola virus disease. http://apps.who.int/iris/bitstream/10665/208883/1/ebolasitrep_10Jun2016_eng pdf?ua=1. Accessed 8 Nov 2016.

Yan, H., & Levs, J. (2014). A worried world watches as Ebola death toll rises; Liberia declares emergency. http://www.cnn.com/2014/08/06/health/africa-ebola-outbreak/index.html. Accessed 11 Aug 2014.

Index